THE
POWER OF
ORGANIC
FITNESS

THE NATURAL WAY TO BE HEALTHIER AND HAPPIER USING FOOD AND LIFESTYLE

COLMAN J. POWER

R^ethink

First published in Great Britain in 2022
by Rethink Press (www.rethinkpress.com)

© Copyright Colman Power

To my mother for raising, feeding and (still) dressing me appropriately for all big social events

To my father for instilling in me a never-give-up attitude and hard work ethic

To my sister for getting me started on my unique path of organic growing

To my little brother, the final member of my immediate family, who was one of the main reasons I came home from Australia to win a country championship with

And to all the people I have surrounded myself with who have had a massive effect on who I have become and helped me become the author of this book

Contents

Introduction

This book is for anyone who is interested in improving their overall health from the moment they get up until the moment they go to bed. It will show you that food has a huge part to play in your overall health and tell you why foods grown in sunlight and a natural environment, without GMO seeds or the harsh chemicals that some people will lead you to believe are the only way to produce enough food to feed the planet, are key to a healthy life. I will stress the importance of buying or growing your own to further improve your health. If you decide to grow your own food, you'll not only get better nutrition; you'll also get free exercise.

Whatever area of your health you are looking to improve, this book will give you the information you need to make the right choices, explaining foods from the ground up and providing you with a simple exercise regime that will maximise your fitness. There is a huge amount of debate about what the best diet is for weight loss or fitness. My preference is for you to understand what food does to the body before jumping on the latest fitness bandwagon or adopting the latest trendy diet. The best diet is the one that suits your lifestyle and matches your fitness goals.

What exactly does the word 'organic' mean, how is it linked to 'gut health', why is fibre so important and how does food affect your mood? These are some of the questions I answer in this book. Huge amounts of research have been done on gut bacteria, much of it at Cork University – only twenty minutes from where I wrote this book. I draw on this and my own master's degree in Organic Horticulture (at the time, Ireland was the only country in Europe offering such a course) to make those answers both authoritative and relevant.

Coming from a country background, having worked on all kinds of farms (from small, organic farms all the way to the opposite end of spectrum – a large, commercial dairy farm with over 3,000 cows where the animals rarely saw direct sunlight not to mention grass, and were fed sprayed non-organic feed and milked three times daily) and now being a fully registered organic grower, I am in an excellent position to assess the many advantages and benefits of organic produce.

I am also a qualified personal trainer and a self-confessed fitness fanatic, so this book is an accumulation of everything I have learned in my career and a distillation of my fascination with how to stay fit and healthy. But it goes beyond that. Health and fitness are closely related to happiness, which is why there is also a chapter on happiness and personal development

For a long time, I struggled to get to grips with my thoughts. A major turning point came when I started to write things down. Truth be told, that's what led to me writing this book. I recognised that my thoughts were not always necessarily unique. It's important to consider that others may have the same challenges as you do. I have shared my thoughts and strategies for achieving happiness and personal development with you in the hope that my experiences and approaches will add value to your life.

With chapters on sleep and the importance of sunlight, as well as exercises and activities for all levels, this book will provide you with a wealth of life tips and traditional wisdom that many of us have lost due to the 'go, go, go!' mentality of the modern world and our loss of connection with nature (which freely provides us with energy-positive sensations if we only know where to look).

Not all foods are created equal and 'cheap' food may not be worth the financial saving. 'You are what you eat' is a common assertion, but as you will learn, no less true for that. The foods we eat have a direct result on how our bodies function. What you eat affects not only your gut, but also your brain. Together, they control your weight and can prevent or eliminate chronic illnesses. By changing how you eat, sleep and exercise, you can completely change the way you look and feel.

After reading this book, you will be in a position to become a fitter, healthier and happier individual. Knowledge is power and this book will give you the power of organic fitness and health. All you have to do is put it into action.

Let's go.

PART ONE
HOW YOUR BODY WORKS

If you belong to a gym, work out at home or exercise at all, you may have heard of macros. Macros are the three main food sources the body runs off: protein, fats and carbohydrates. Every food item we consume can be broken down into carbohydrates, protein or fats. Understanding your individual macro requirements is important and these depend on your height, weight and activity level. Balancing and manipulating macros is essential if you are looking to lose weight or gain lean muscle.

Reading food labels and using fitness apps in order to achieve that balance is important, but the thing about food labels is that they don't tell you the chemical content of what you are eating. The body runs more efficiently when there are fewer toxins and processes involved in the food we eat. The more chemicals we consume, the more work the body has to do to break down and eliminate them, leaving less energy for the day's essential activities. This is one of the reasons why I recommend organic food throughout this book.

In Part One, I advise you on the best possible intake of foods that are either a protein, a fat or carbohydrate and how you can get them from local and chemical-free sources.

1
Carbs And Protein

In this first chapter, I look at the first two macros: carbohydrates and protein. Fats will be discussed in Chapter 2. The number of calories we need each day depends on our height, weight and activity level. To start with, here is a handy summary of the comparative calorific value of the three macros:

Macros	Calories
Carbohydrates	4 calories per gram
Protein	4 calories per gram
Fats	9 calories per gram

Types of carbs

Carbohydrates, commonly known as carbs, are sugar molecules. When we eat carbs, they are digested and broken down into glycogen, which is either used directly as fuel or stored as glucose in the muscles.

Carbs are often given a bad name because too many will lead to weight gain. It's true that the glucose stored in the muscles after we eat carbs holds on to water, which can make the numbers on a scale increase. Carbs also cause spikes in blood sugar, which can prompt hunger cravings, but they are the body's primary source of energy for the brain and muscles. For optimal health, it is important to find the right carbs, matching activity levels to carbohydrate consumption, and not avoid them completely.

There are two main types of carbohydrates: complex carbohydrates and simple carbohydrates.

Complex carbohydrates

Complex carbohydrates are exactly that: complex. They take longer to be broken down by the body, giving a slower release of energy and stabilising your blood sugar levels for steady energy levels. It's the fibre in these foods that makes them harder for the body to break down. (This will be discussed in Chapter 3 on gut health.)

Complex carbohydrates that I recommend are wholemeal breads, including sourdough bread, brown pasta, oats and flour, quinoa and bulgur wheat, beans, lentils and any vegetable (all organic of course).

Simple carbohydrates

Simple carbohydrates are more easily digested by the body, giving you a quick release of their energy and a spike in your blood sugar levels. Examples of simple carbs are fruits or refined carbohydrates such as white pasta or white rice.

Neither type of carbohydrate source is good or bad in itself. The important thing is to incorporate them into your diet at different times during the day to maximise their benefit. For example, if you want a quick release of energy before intense exercise, a sports event or need a pick-me-up, a shot of simple carbohydrates will give your body a spike in blood sugar levels that would be desirable at that time.

Processed foods

We live in an age where 'ready meals' wrapped in shiny plastic are too easily available. Processed foods are high in carbs. What's more, when a food item is processed, some of its beneficial properties are removed. As a general rule, the more something is processed, the less beneficial it is likely to be. Take, for example, breakfast cereals that are made from processed wheat. Sugar is then added, along with a whole host of stabilisers and preservatives to stop the cereal going off. The manufacturers may advertise that they are fortified with vitamins during the processing stage, but it is rather like putting a dress on a pig: it's still a pig.

Another example is white rice. This is rice that has had its outer layer removed (which is where valuable minerals and fibres such as B vitamins, iron and zinc are contained). Cheap grain is also typically sprayed with harsh chemicals, which are endocrine- and hormone-disruptors. The same applies to white bread. When you eat white bread, the body quickly breaks it down to give you a rapid increase in energy, but when your blood sugar levels drop again, there is a drop in energy, a slump in mood, and in some cases, headaches. This is why brown, wholemeal bread is preferable. It contains that added layer on the grain (which gives it its colour), as well as added fibre and B6 vitamins (which help produce the 'happy hormone' serotonin), manganese (used for digesting protein) and magnesium (which aids in relaxing the muscles). There are similar benefits to choosing brown rice over white, so choose whole grains over polished ones for a healthier version of you.

Knowing what foods are more or less processed can be tricky, but if a food comes with no ingredient list (like a whole head of broccoli), you're on to a winner, especially when it's organic. Minimising processed foods such as crackers, breakfast cereal bars, sweet-ened cakes or breads and sauces with added sugar are vital for preventing a rollercoaster spike in blood sugar levels. Instead, choose whole foods such as brown sourdough bread, whole grains (oats, brown pasta, quinoa, bulgur wheat), vegetables, beans, len-tils and fruits with a high fibre content. This is why I am a major fan of single-ingredient foods.

Benefits of eating less processed food

A reduction in processed foods and an increase of whole foods will always be beneficial. These benefits typically include fewer chemicals, a lower calorie count and a higher nutrient content. With whole foods – ie, foods in a more natural state – we get a vast array of nutrients acting together. In the case of carbs, mini-mally processed carbohydrates are preferable over processed or refined carbohydrates for the following reasons:

- Greater fibre intake
- Enhanced satiety (you stay fuller for longer)
- Controlled blood sugar levels (see below)

It's true that whole foods can seems less flavoursome than processed foods. The key to making them taste nice is to invest in a spice rack, with each spice bring-ing additional health benefits (see Chapter 8).

Fruit, fructose and sugar

The main difference between fruit and vegetables is that vegetables have much lower levels of sugar. Fruits and vegetables are nutrient-dense food sources which also contain fibre. Leafy green vegetables are low in calories and ridiculously hard to overeat. I've never heard anyone say, 'It was all that broccoli that made me gain weight!'

Sugar is a carbohydrate, which is why some diets demonise fruit. Its natural sugar, fructose, is thought to lead to weight gain. Admittedly, fructose can be converted into glucose pretty easily and lead to weight gain if eaten to excess, but it can balance blood sugar levels if eaten at certain times, eg, directly after training. The main benefit that fructose in whole fruit has over other sugars is its fibre, which prevents a spike in our blood sugar levels, with the added advantage of improving our gut health. Fruits also contain a host of vitamins, minerals, antioxidants, and fibre. Most importantly, they curb a sweet tooth.

When choosing fruits, always eat them in their whole form, when they are in season, and organic – as nature designed. Some fruits such as dates, grapes and mangoes contain pure glucose, which gives your body less work to do, leading to an increase in energy.

Don't be afraid of fruit. Use it to your advantage, eating it in the morning or after a workout, for example.

I love fruit. Typically, I eat fruit in the morning with oats, flaxseeds and a protein source. I have fruit again after I work out – another time when the body needs carbohydrates. I recommend this approach to people who are not only looking to lose weight, but are also seeking increased energy. Foods containing carbs give us energy, so we must use this energy before we can tap into our reserve fat stores. In other words, you must first use your glycogen (stored carbs in your muscles) before you can use your body fat as a direct energy source. Fruit should be one of the last things removed from your diet. Fruit is the rarely the problem; processed foods are.

Blood sugar levels

We have mentioned 'balancing blood sugar levels', which is a term often used by health professionals, but what does it really mean and how does it affect your health and fitness? Blood sugar is, quite simply, the amount of sugar in the blood. Our blood sugar rises whenever we eat, but the pace at which it rises, and how high it rises, depends on the food item.

As we can see from the graph below, carbohydrates have the greatest effect on blood sugar levels, followed to a significantly lesser extent by protein and then fats. After looking at this graph, you might decide to take out carbohydrates from your diet altogether, but this would make your food choices extremely difficult as carbs are found in breads, grains, vegetables and even desserts. Besides, if you have low blood sugar levels, you will have low energy levels. Finding balance is key to whatever diet you choose.

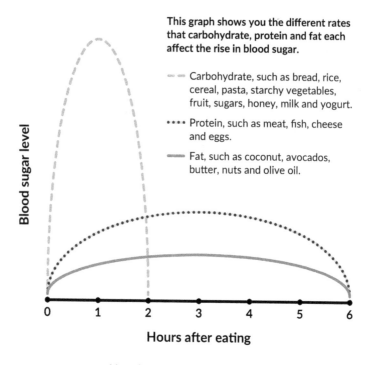

This graph shows you the different rates that carbohydrate, protein and fat each affect the rise in blood sugar.

– – Carbohydrate, such as bread, rice, cereal, pasta, starchy vegetables, fruit, sugars, honey, milk and yogurt.

•••• Protein, such as meat, fish, cheese and eggs.

━━ Fat, such as coconut, avocados, butter, nuts and olive oil.

How food affects blood sugar

It is also important to remember that the different types of carbs (simple and complex) affect blood sugar levels differently. Eating white bread, white pasta and sugar, for example, will cause blood sugar spikes, whereas eating brown bread, wholemeal pasta and fruit will lead to a more gradual blood sugar increase. As a general rule, the less processed or sweet something is, the less of an effect it will have on your blood sugar levels. Jumping from low to high blood sugar levels is like riding a roller coaster: one minute you're down, then you're up – and what goes up fast, comes down fast (which is OK if it's a roller coaster ride you're on, but not something you want going on in your blood).

Foods increase your blood sugar levels and insulin decreases them. Insulin is produced when blood sugar goes up. Insulin's job is to take out sugar from the bloodstream and put it in the cells – first to the muscle cells, next the liver cells, and finally, the fat cells. Incidentally, this emphasises the advantage of having muscle: you can store more energy. When your blood sugar levels are balanced, it helps with brain function and food cravings and prevents mood swings (hangry is a real thing), so how can we control them?

How to balance your blood sugar levels

- **Reduce processed foods:** If food is less processed, it will take the body longer to digest it and produce less of a spike in blood sugar. The excessive amounts of pesticides commonly sprayed on non-organic produce can also lead to insulin resistance.[1]

- **Balance your meals:** When we consume foods in combination, we get the benefit of protein and fats slowing down the absorption of glucose into the bloodstream. Simple meals such as sweet potatoes, kale, pumpkin seeds, kidney beans and Brussels sprouts with a spice like curry powder, a dollop of yoghurt and sprinkled with hemp seeds are balanced and well-rounded. Sweet potatoes are a complex carb, pumpkin seeds are a healthy fat, kidney beans and yoghurt are the protein sources, while hemp seeds also add protein and healthy fats. All these foods come with their own micronutrients too: sweet potatoes have vitamin A (good for skin health), pumpkin seeds have zinc (good for immune system), kidney beans have magnesium (can reduce anxiety), spices are full of antioxidants and reduce stress on the body and yoghurt has protein and calcium (as well as being a natural probiotic). Balancing your meals provides diversity in your diet, which means improved overall health.

- **Eat regularly:** When you eat at regular intervals, you are preventing an extreme low that can lead to overeating in the next meal. That common feeling of being bloated and having reduced brain power that can lead to being unproductive will also be avoided. The overeating of carbohydrates is common after a long interval and will lead to an unwanted store of body fat and increase the production of insulin in the body, leading to a dip in blood sugar. Eating at least one meal of the day with low (or no) carbs and bumping up on your dark, leafy greens and high-protein foods with healthy fats instead is the answer.

- **Exercise regularly:** Walking 10,000 steps a day, running, weight training or doing fitness classes all reduce sugar in the blood. This not only helps you to control your blood sugars, but also helps you prevent weight gain. If you work out with weights such as dumbbells at home or in the gym, you get the added advantage of changing your body composition, killing two birds with one stone. Another advantage of exercise is that you deplete the glycogen levels in your body, which will improve your insulin sensitivity so that you can fuel up on carbs for a boost of energy without excess amounts being stored in reserve as body fat. This is why I eat the bulk of my carbs after I work out.

Protein

Protein is the second of the three essential macronutrients that must be part of our diet. Protein is often thought of as food for those who go to the gym or want to build muscle, but protein has many functions in the body – it's not just for building muscle. Certainly, protein has to be consumed with any fitness goal, but protein also keeps you fuller for longer, improves your skin health, stabilises your blood sugar levels, regulates your hunger hormones and helps maintain the muscle you have when you are trying to lose weight (it repairs cells that we tear during exercise). Protein also supplies the body's essential amino acids (see below). If there was a tablet that could do all that, we all would be taking it!

TOP TIP

Most people don't hit their daily protein target. A general rule is to aim for 30 grams per main meal. This doesn't have to come from a single source (eg, a single chicken breast). You can have several different protein sources for more benefits, but every meal should focus on a protein source.

Amino acids

Amino acids are the 'building blocks' of proteins and play many critical roles in your body, including the synthesis of hormones and neurotransmitters. There are nine essential amino acids: histidine, isoleucine, leucine, lysine, methionine, phenylalanine, threonine, tryptophan and valine. These are labelled as essential because the body cannot make them, so we must absorb them from our diet.

Thermic effect

Another advantage protein has over the other two macronutrients, especially if your goal is weight loss, is what's known as the 'thermic effect'. If you guessed that 'thermo' has something to do with temperature, you're right. The thermic (or thermogenic) effect (also called diet-induced thermogenesis) is the increase in your metabolism above its normal rate from the processing of food. The higher your metabolism is, the more calories you burn, making it easier to lose weight and keep it off.

When it comes to calories, not all foods are equal, so choosing the right diet is not a simple matter of counting calories. The diagram below shows the amount of energy used in the breakdown of each macronutrient.

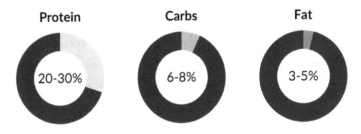

The amount of energy used in the breakdown of each macronutrient

As you can see, protein foods use far more calories than either carbs or fats as they are broken down: because of the thermic effect, protein ends up having 70% useable calories. This raises your body's core temperature – which is another reason to eat protein foods in each meal, especially for weight management.

Digesting and breaking down foods being such a huge process that the body must go through, eating the right type of protein is key. Protein tends to be associated with meat, but you don't have to eat meat to get protein into your diet. There are also many plant-based protein sources.

Plant-based protein sources

Meat, fish, dairy, poultry and other animal produce contains the nine essential amino acids that we must consume in our diet, so these are known as complete protein sources. Plant-based sources of protein are typically short of one or more of the essential amino acids, but there are a few complete, plant-based protein sources. These are what vegans and vegetarians must eat to have optimal health (although you don't have to be one to eat them!). The five food items shown in the table below contain all nine essential amino acids – with added fibre, of course:

	Suggested serving size	Total protein
Tempeh	100 g	18 g
Quinoa	100 g	14 g
Tofu	100 g	13 g
Bulgur wheat	100 g	12 g
Hemp seeds	15 g	5 g

Note: 100 grams of tofu or tempeh is about the size of your fist and 15 grams of hemp seeds is a big spoonful.

Plant-based protein is typically lower in protein than meat sources, but also typically lower in calories, so we can eat more and stay the same weight. If you want to add more plant-based foods to your diet, eating higher-protein meals is necessary to maintain the muscle you currently have as well as keeping you fuller for longer, which helps if you are trying to lose weight. Unlike meat, plant-based protein has the added advantage of also being a source of fibre.

TOP TIP

Don't be fooled into thinking you are eating healthily with meat substitutes such as Quorn. These have ingredient lists longer than the Bayeux Tapestry, with added preservatives and poor-quality fats all wrapped in plastic and shipped in from miles away. Single-ingredient, complete proteins are what you are looking for if you are trying to be healthier.

Soya (or soy) is also a high-quality protein source, though it also contains a fair amount of carbs. When choosing soya-based products, reach for organic that does not use GMO seeds and know that it is not only beneficial for you but also the soil.

Oestrogen in soya

Soya-based products such as tempeh and tofu are often thought to increase levels of oestrogen in the body, which affects a woman's hormone balance and reduces testosterone in men. Soya does contain a high concentration of isoflavones – a type of plant oestrogen (phytoestrogen) that is similar in function to human oestrogen – but with much weaker effects. It should also be considered that far more hormonal harm is caused by the harsh chemicals applied to non-organic produce. In any case, a diet of kale, spinach, spring onions, beetroot and pumpkin seeds (which naturally increase testosterone in men) will give you more than enough fibre to bind to excess hormones and toxins in the body so that you will pass them out.

Incomplete protein sources

Peas, beans, nuts and grains are also sources of protein, but 'incomplete sources' because they lack some of the essential amino acids and also contain carbs. They can, however, be combined with foods such as pasta, which provide the essential amino acids that we must consume from our diet. Nuts also contain healthy fats (see Chapter 2).

One of my favourite protein sources is lentils, which are high in beta carotene, an antioxidant that can improve your skin colour. Antioxidants neutralise free radicals that cause stress on the body, and less stress is more success, especially regarding your health. Lentils combined with kidney beans and sprinkled with pink Himalayan salt and your favourite greens make up a complete protein meal. (Note: when you start eating more single-ingredient foods, you'll need more salt in your diet.)

Combining two or more incomplete protein sources can compensate for any lack of amino acids in individual sources. For example, grains are low in the amino acid lysine, and beans and nuts (legumes) are low in methionine. When grains and legumes are eaten together (such as rice and beans, or peanut butter on wholewheat, sourdough bread), they form a complete protein that has all nine essential amino acids. The chart below makes it easy to visualise how to make complete proteins from incomplete, plant-based sources:

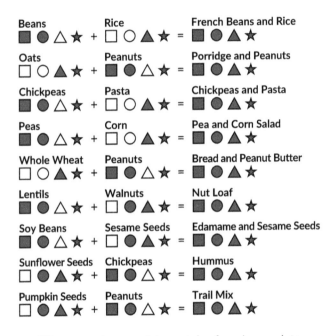

Ways to make complete proteins from incomplete plant-based sources

TOP TIP

When combining foods to give you the protein you need, you don't have to put them together in a single meal, like chickpeas and rice (though that is another good match). As long as you consume it the same day, everything will be broken down in your gut *anyway*.

Animal-based protein sources

Fish, meats, eggs and other dairy products are all high-protein foods. There are both pros and cons to consuming meat and dairy products. Meat is nutrient-dense, with easily absorbed iron and vitamin B12, which affects your energy levels, as iron carries oxygen around the body. Yoghurts and cheese can be beneficial if your body can tolerate the lactose in the milk products, as they can naturally improve your gut health (see Chapter 3). Eggs are nature's multivitamin and something that I have eaten since the age of eighteen (when I started taking responsibility for my diet), though I now consume them in a slightly different way. Like Rocky, I used to drink three raw eggs after a workout, which was my equivalent to a protein shake without the added sugar. With my knowledge of nutrition (and improved culinary skills), I now cook my eggs and take a four-ingredient, plant-based protein supplement after whole foods to hit my daily protein target.

Any meat or dairy products are best eaten organic. This will prevent excess antibiotics and growth hormones getting into your body, as these are prohibited in registered organic meat products. Organically raised animals must be grass-fed, where all the natural vitamins come from the soil. (You will find more examples of protein sources that you can and should consume in Part Two of this book.)

Summary

The health and fitness industry has marketed protein supplements so well that we have forgotten where protein originally comes from. I hope this chapter has clarified that and given you an understanding of the relative importance of carbohydrates and protein in your diet. This understanding is essential because any food – protein, fat or carbohydrate – affects the body the moment you consume it. This is the subject of Chapter 4 on gut health, but first let's look at that most misunderstood of the three macros: fats.

2
Fats

Fats are an essential part of any diet. They contribute to the taste and the texture of foods, from the smoothness of avocados to the crunch of an almond, or nut butters (though if you prefer smooth over crunchy, we can't be friends). Fats are also a major source of energy and a critical component of cells and tissues. They aid in the absorption of vital fat-soluble vitamins, improve skin health and increase brain function. In short, fats are essential for optimal health.

More often than not we have a negative connection to the word 'fat'. This is mostly because we have heard that if you eat fat, you will get fat, which is not entirely correct. There are, of course, different types of fats and certain types of fat will make you fat. Adding the right fats into your diet is key.

Fats differ from the other two macronutrients (carbs and protein – see Chapter 1) in one main respect: they contain 9 calories per gram, whereas carbohydrates and protein contain only 4 calories per gram. To put that in perspective, 100 grams of nut butter is nearly 600 calories (because it is made up of protein, fats and some carbs), while 100 grams of chicken breast is only 88 calories.

There are four main types of fat: saturated fats, mono-unsaturated fats, polyunsaturated fats and trans-fatty acids. Almost all foods that contain fat have a balance of two or more types of fats. Let's look at each of these in turn.

Saturated fats

These fats are generally solid at room temperature and typically come from animal food products. The use of saturated fats has both positive and negative aspects, so foods that contain it should not be automatically demonised. Studies have found saturated fats to be both beneficial and harmful (not in the same study, of course).[2] It's always best to make up your own mind and look to your specific situation. Each food item is not just made up of one thing. It has benefits, but may have negative effects if over-consumed, which give rise to an unbalanced lifestyle.

The benefits of foods that contain saturated fats is they have all nine essential amino acids, omega-3 and omega-6, vitamin B12 and a high iron content. There are certainly some products containing saturated fats (eg, meats, eggs, soya products and coconut oil) which, if excessively consumed, can have negative effects – like almost any food. In the case of saturated fat, you *can* have too much of a good thing. If you do eat meat and eggs, make sure they are from grass-fed, organic sources to maximise their benefits to you.

Frying with vegetable and coconut oil

Oils are high in calories, as they are mostly fat and have little of the other two macronutrients, protein or carbs, which is why they are often said to be bad for you. What is not well known is that saturated fats are found in vegetable oil, which is typically used in the frying of food in restaurants and cafes because it is cheap. The heating, cooling and reheating of vegetable oil causes the oil to oxidise, and excess oxidation speeds up ageing in the body and can cause inflammation, leading to poor skin health, and on a more serious level, chronic illness. It pays to know what oil is being used if you dine out (although fried foods are not exactly what I'm recommending in this book).

Instead of frying with oil, especially if you're watching your waistline, I recommend cooking with vegetable stock and water. Certain saturated fats such as coconut oil have gained popularity due to their ability to improve cognitive function, as well as being suitable for cooking at high temperatures, which is why

I always keep coconut oil within reach for my pan frying.

Foods containing saturated fats

The most common foods that contain saturated fats are:

- Fatty red meat (eg, beef and lamb)
- Coconut milk and flesh
- Dairy butter
- Cheese
- Cream
- Yoghurt (milk-based)
- Coconut oil
- Vegetable oil

Mono-unsaturated fats

Mono-unsaturated fats are generally liquid at room temperature. They support insulin sensitivity and weight loss and can increase energy levels and speed up recovery from an injury or a workout. Mono-unsaturated fats also have anti-inflammatory properties. Like saturated fats, they contain 9 calories per gram.

Monounsaturated fats are found in all meats, but not all meat is created equally and you should always buy organic meat from grass-fed animals. One of the aims of this book, however, is to persuade you to eat more plant-based foods, which provide added benefits: fibre, more antioxidants, easier digestion and typically lower calories. Examples of foods containing mono-unsaturated fats are:

- Avocados
- Brazil nuts
- Egg yolks
- Nuts (almonds, cashews, hazelnuts, peanuts, pistachios) and their butters and oils
- Meats
- Olive oil

Frying with olive oil

Organic extra virgin olive oil is my favourite cooking oil for many reasons – taste being one. Olive oil has a good omega-3 to -6 ratio (see below), it has a medium to high smoke-point, it's packed full of vitamin E and has a type of antioxidant called oleocanthal.

To get good olive oil, first make sure it is organic and comes from a single source of olives such as a family-run business (all of which can be found from reading the label or by a quick web search.) It is also best to buy olive oil that is in a dark bottle, as it will go off over time. Olive oil is not like wine; it doesn't improve with age. That's why I have some every day, either sautéing my vegetables in a pan or cooking my eggs in it.

Polyunsaturated fats

The prefix 'poly' comes from Greek and means 'many'. And polyunsaturated fats have two or more carbon-double bonds, which in plain English means that, in the right amounts, they improve blood flow, skin condition, muscle repair and brain function.

There are two main types of polyunsaturated fats: omega-3 and omega-6. Both omega-6 and omega-3 fats are needed for brain function, as the brain is made up of 60-70% fats. This is why you might hear of people taking omega-3 fish oil supplements before exams. (If you've ever been called a fathead, you should take it as a compliment!) Both omega-3 and omega-6 fats must be absorbed from our diet as the body cannot make them.

Omega-6

Omega-6 is needed in the body for muscle function as well as to stimulate healthy skin and hair development. Omega-6 can also cause inflammation. Inflammation is often seen as a negative, but it is part of the body's natural response to stress. When you twist your ankle or knee, for example, your body sends fluid to that area to protect it, which is the first process of healing. We need a certain amount of inflammation, but not too much, as excessive fats from oils and food items can increase inflammation in the body and lead to facial spots. Excessive amounts of inflammation require anti-inflammatory assistance. Medication is often recommended, but the best medicine is the right food, especially if it's organic.

Ideally, we need a ratio of 4:1 omega-6 to omega-3. As omega-6 is found in sunflower oil, rapeseed oil and corn oil (which are typically used in the preserving of processed foods), as well as in meats and nuts, a 'standard' diet typically provides sufficient omega-6 (or even too much, which can lead to the problem of achieving a healthy 4:1 ratio).

Omega-3

It is important to consume omega-3-rich food, as most foods, whether meat- or plant-based, contain higher amounts of omega-6 than omega-3. On the other hand, organic food has higher amounts of omega-3, as omega is found in the soil (yet another reason to eat organic food).

Omega-3 fats increase the protein made in the body called brain-derived neurotrophic factor (BDNF), which promotes the brain's ability to create new memory cells and can enhance your mood. Omega-3 also helps to reduce inflammation, dilates the blood vessels, improves the body's use of carbohydrates and increases insulin sensitivity so that the body can use glucose, our main source of energy, more effectively. The main reasons for consuming omega-3-rich foods are because they:

1. **Reduce inflammation:** Inflammation occurs when we cause damage to any cell, whether through a cut or wound, by tearing muscle fibres during exercise, when we have an infection or disease or if there are excess toxins in our food. By eating omega-3-rich foods, especially chemical-free ones, we can increase recovery time by reducing muscle soreness and prevent chronic diseases that occur due to excessive inflammation in the body. These range from asthma and eczema to arthritis and cancer.

2. **Dilate blood vessels:** Dilation of blood vessels increases the flow of blood to the heart, muscles and brain, reducing fatigue and giving you more energy. When you have more energy, you are more productive; and when you are more productive, you're likely to get paid more! Greater levels of blood flow also reduce blockages, helping to prevent heart problems. Who doesn't want to think clearer, improve their training and get paid more for being more productive at work?

Omega-3 fats can be split up into:

1. Alpha-linolenic acid (ALA), found in flaxseeds, walnuts, chia seeds and hemp seeds.

2. Docosahexaenoic acid (DHA) and eicosapentaenoic acid (EPA), found in micro-algae (so in fish like mackerel, salmon and sardines). Eggs, meat and greens also have some DHA, but lesser amounts than sea creatures.

Our body can convert ALA to DHA and EPA, but not all of the plant sources of omega-3 are converted by the body, so vegetarians (and especially vegans) may have to supplement. Here are some omega-3-rich foods to add to your diet:

- Fish (especially oily fish or cod-liver)

- Chia seeds

- Flax and hemp seeds (my favourite)

- Sunflower seeds

- Walnuts

Flax seed oil has about the highest omega-3 content of any cooking oil, with a low smoke-point. It's also ideal for drizzling over salads.

Fish fats

Fish are a good way of getting both omega-6, and particularly omega-3, fats. Salmon, mackerel and sardines are the fish with the highest polyunsaturated fat content, but increasing your intake of omega-3 is unfortunately not as simple as eating more fish – for a number of reasons.

First, the way fish have been reared affects the amount of healthy fats they contain. Wild salmon and other free-roaming fish are best. They eat smaller sea creatures that contain omega-3, while farmed fish don't get the same food sources and don't have as much room to roam, which also leads to lower levels of omega-3. Sea fish can still contain toxins such as micro-plastics due to pollution, so your best option is to buy your fish fresh from a local supplier or catch some yourself. We cannot reverse the pollution we have done to our oceans, but we can reduce the amount of toxins we consume. A rule of thumb is: the closer you go to the source, the better (which also applies to fruits and vegetables). Knowing where your food comes from, regardless of which diet you choose, is essential.

The omega-3 from plant sources is more difficult for the body to break down to a useable form, so meat sources are often recommended first, but just because something is difficult doesn't mean you shouldn't do it. The trick is to eat fats that have a good omega-3 to -6 ratio, like organic, free-range pasture-raised eggs. For breakfast, try an oats, kale and flax seed smoothie; for lunch, a spinach and boiled egg salad with peppers, cucumbers, tomatoes and kidney beans, plus cayenne pepper and hemp seeds; and for dinner, any high-protein food with spinach, lentils, onions, garlic and walnuts all in a stir-fry with organic vegetable stock. My mouth is watering already!

TOP TIP

Even healthy fats contain around 9 calories per gram so remember that they must still be consumed in moderation and relative to your height and weight.

Healthy fats in organic meat and eggs

There is scientific evidence that organic meat, eggs and other dairy produce have higher amounts of omega-3 than their 'conventional' equivalents. This is due to the use of natural feed in the raising of free-range, pasture-grazed animals, which consume a larger amount of nutrients from their feed. When animals are raised using conventional methods, antibiotics and excessive amounts of harsh chemicals can be applied to the land the animals feed on.[3]

Trans fatty acids

Trans fatty acids are fats (mostly vegetable oils) that have been chemically modified to make them more hydrogenated, which means that they can be used to prolong the shelf life of processed foods. Essentially, hydrogen molecules are added to the oils. Because trans fatty acids are man-made, the body cannot break them down, which has all kinds of negative consequences.

First, as we have seen, vegetable oils are high in omega-6, which can cause excess inflammation in the body, pushing the omega-3 to -6 ratio in the wrong direction. Using these oils can also lead to weight gain, poor skin health and diabetes. Trans fatty acids lower your good cholesterol (HDL) and increase your bad cholesterol (LDL), leading to heart problems later in life. Examples of products that typically contain trans fatty acids are:

- Fried foods (eg, chips, burgers, sausages, breaded chicken)

- Cakes and pastries

- Biscuits

- Doughnuts

- Crackers

- Cereal bars

- Microwave popcorn

- Protein bars

- Pizzas (especially frozen)

How can you avoid consuming trans fatty acids? At home, use organic olive or coconut oils instead of vegetable oils or margarine and eat whole foods. When eating out, choose foods that are baked, grilled or steamed, rather than fried. Skip those shop-bought pizzas for alternatives, or make your own using organic flour, local tomatoes that you know are chemical-free (ideally home-grown) and organic cheese. Mmm...

Summary

With an ever-changing environment, animals have a role to play in the cycle of nutrients through their manure, particularly on organic farms. Whether you are a big meat eater or not, these food sources contain vital minerals and vitamins for optimal health. For example, the iron found in red meat is more easily absorbed than the iron in plants and will benefit individuals who have a low iron level and who would otherwise tend to lack energy. The same applies to vitamin B12, which is needed to make protein, to carry oxygen (essential for increased energy levels) and for a healthy nervous system. Vitamin B12 is found in all meat and fish sources as well as dairy products such as cheese and eggs. Vegans must consume vitamin

B12 from fortified food sources such as soya products, plant milks and yeast flakes (which, to some people, taste like cheese). Fish, meats and eggs are also a quick and sure way of getting your essential amino acids.

The essential point to remember is that organic produce is free from antibiotics and excessive amounts of harsh chemicals, so by all means, include organic chicken, beef, eggs and wild-caught fish in your diet. I believe that animals should be used to fertilise the land and live happy healthy lives, which happens on small, local organic farms, so support them as much as you can.

3
Gut Health

The gut starts at the mouth, travelling south to the oesophagus, then the stomach and into the small intestine, and finally, to the large intestine (also known as the colon). If your gut health is not what it should be, this affects the whole body, so in this chapter I will explain the signs of poor gut health and give you ways to improve it. (More details of this are available on my YouTube channel.)

Gut health has become a popular topic over the last twenty years. Studies have linked good gut health with improved immune system, nervous system, skin condition,[4] mood and mental health,[5] and to the avoidance of weight gain and chronic diseases – in other words, with overall health and wellbeing. When you are told that you should 'go with your gut', it's for a very good reason.

There are a tremendous number of micro-organisms inside you – trillions of them to be exact – and others are found on the surface of various parts of the body such as your skin. These micro-organisms (also known as microbiota) may be tiny, but they make up for their lack of size by their sheer numbers. If you were to weigh your entire micro-organism population, it would be as heavy as your brain, totalling 2-3 pounds (around 1 kilogram).

These micro-organisms are affected by your surroundings, which is why if you sit at a desk for eight hours a day, you need to get outside. A high percentage of micro-organisms are located on the largest organ of your body, your skin, so exposing your skin to the air gives you more diverse microbiota (a good reason to go for that Sunday hike in shorts and a T-shirt). Beneficial micro-organisms travel in the wind and are deposited on leaves or any living material, which means that it's the living materials in nature that improve your health inside and out with every breath you take and every bite you eat. Another large percentage of these tiny little guys live in the foods you eat, which is why I am writing about them in this book.

Signs of an unhealthy gut

An unhealthy gut can be caused by, or be the result of:

1. Food intolerances

2. Chronic stress

3. Bloating

4. Eating a highly processed diet

5. Constant fatigue

6. Poor sleep

Food intolerances

Food intolerances are the result of certain foods causing unpleasant symptoms such as rashes or blushing of the skin, bloating, gas, stomach pain, diarrhoea and nausea. Food intolerance is not the same as a food allergy (although they can have some of the same symptoms), so it is important to speak to a doctor if you suspect that you have food intolerance.

Determining which foods you are intolerant of is difficult, but it can be done with an elimination diet. This is where you progressively remove common foods that may cause bloating: dairy, legumes or beans, excess meats and even some vegetables. Keep a food diary and look for patterns. Better still, work with a trained nutritionist to prevent nutritional deficiency during this process.

Chronic stress

We all have a certain amount of stress in our lives, but when it builds up, it can lead to chronic stress. Chronic stress is hard on your whole body, including your gut. It's impossible to eliminate stress, but reducing it is vital. Here are some ways I deal with stress:

- Walking

- Bathing in Epsom salts

- Eating high-magnesium foods such as greens, beans, legumes and cacao (organic, of course, as organic produce has more antioxidants, which increase blood flow and reduce stress, see Chapter 7)

- Reducing phone time

- Grounding and stretching, with deep nasal breathing (see Chapter 10)

- Training. This temporarily increases stress, but makes you more relaxed afterwards, so that you sleep better (see Chapter 11)

All these things also have knock-on health benefits. For example, when you improve your food choices, your energy levels increase. When you have more energy, you are much more likely to train... These are all simple things to incorporate into your day. It's easy to say, 'I don't have time for them,' but if you really don't, then you not only have a stress issue, you also likely have a time management issue. Make some of these fit your day.

Bloating

You wouldn't believe how common bloating is. Chewing your food is the first process of the digestive system. If you decide to have your lunch on the go at your desk with your phone in hand or just wolf it down, the chances are you are not chewing it enough. The American gastroenterologist, nutritionist and author, William John Bulsiewicz, recommends chewing your food at least forty times.[6] Try counting now and then to see how much (or how little) you are chewing your food. My eating habits have changed over the years. I have gradually slowed down and become more mindful of the food I am eating, which makes me enjoy food even more as well as having other benefits. It has helped me improve my overall health, including my gut health, resulting in a better mood, reduced bloating and fewer 'alien' sounds coming from my stomach area.

It also increases the signals to the brain to release more of the satiating hormone, leptin, which tells you that you've eaten enough and prevents you overeating. Think of it like this: if we don't start the digestive process well, we are playing catch-up for the rest of it, leading to unnecessary stress on the body. Here are some tips to improve the digestive process and reduce bloating:

- Put your fork down between bites

- Count the number of times you chew to see how close you are to forty

- Eat with a small spoon. (This one is a new favourite of mine.) You would not believe how much this helps by preventing you from scoffing and wondering why you're hungry all the time

When you practice these methods, you will soon feel that you've eaten enough, so not only does chewing your food thoroughly help reduce bloating – it's also a top weight loss tip!

Highly processed diet

By now, I'm sure you are aware that processed foods are not recommended. There are many reasons for this, but one that is relevant here is that processed foods are typically soft (cakes, buns, soft cheeses, etc) and therefore require little chewing. Anything that doesn't take a lot of effort to chew has less fibre, which your gut microbes miss out on. Processed foods like refined breakfast cereals, sugar-filled biscuits, cakes or desserts have also been linked to increased inflammation in the body.[7]

Processed foods are also more often than not loaded with sugar, which decreases the amount of good gut bacteria and increases the bad bacteria. This imbalance can lead to increased sugar cravings, which can damage your gut. High amounts of refined sugars, particularly high-fructose corn syrup, are typically found in sweetened yoghurts, a common lunchtime snack. My healthy tip for this is to buy plain yoghurt (dairy, soya or coconut) and add berries or seasonal fruit (all organic, of course). This provides added fibre and natural sweetness.

Constant fatigue

If you have energy imbalances or say, 'I'm always tired,' this is a sure sign that your engine is not running smoothly. The gut is the main driver of the body, as it breaks down the food we eat into energy we can use (dependent on the fuel we feed it, of course). The body's first source of energy is carbohydrates (see Chapter 1). Complex carbohydrates are preferable, as these types of foods have added fibre, which feeds your gut the essential micro-organisms. When we eat complex carbs, our microbes naturally multiply and increase the breakdown of the nutrients in that food item as well as the combination of other foods we eat during the day.

My top recommendation for complex carbs is – you guessed it – fresh, raw organic vegetables. These are packed not only full of fibre (a type of carbohydrate that your gut feeds on), but also with a host of nutrients, including iron, magnesium, B vitamins and antioxidants, to name a few. Another of my favourites is brown, whole-grain sourdough bread, not only for the added fibre, but also because its fermentation aids gut health. You can either buy sourdough bread at local farmers' markets or bake your own.

Poor sleep

Poor sleep is often a result of an unhealthy gut due to a poor diet. The majority of the body's serotonin is produced in the gut and this hormone affects mood and sleep. Having a fibre-filled meal in the evening will increase the production of serotonin in the body before you go to sleep, but it is also important to not eat too close to bedtime as this may also affect your sleep (see Chapter 11).

Having a diverse gut microbiome can also give you a better night's sleep. The more diverse the fibre in your diet, the better your body will function and the better you'll sleep. Aim to consume over twenty different plants throughout the week, ranging from salads, spinach, kale, beetroot, beans, peas, peppers, tomatoes, carrots, parsnips, onions, leeks and tubers to grains. This will not only improve your sleep, but also increase your intake of fibre, vitamins, minerals and antioxidants.[8]

Five ways to improve gut health

I have already suggested some things *not to do* so that you don't suffer the effects of poor gut health. Here are some positive ways to improve your gut health:

1. Eat more whole grains

2. Limit artificial sweeteners

3. Incorporate more prebiotics in your diet

4. Incorporate probiotics in your diet

5. Eat organic produce

Eat more whole grains

Whole grains should be a staple in your diet. They have not had their outer coating stripped of the fibrous husk and bran (hence their name). Whole grains are typically a good source of non-heme iron, magnesium, phosphorus and fibre, which is why they're in this section of the book. Iron in food comes in two forms: heme and non-heme. Non-heme iron typically comes from plant sources and is less easily absorbed by the body than heme iron, which is found in meat and animal products.

I particularly recommend organic oats, which have been a staple in my diet in for a long time. I typically consume them either in an oat smoothie or after they have been steeped overnight in maca and cacao and with a host of nuts, seeds and organic eggs. There are gluten-free oats, too. (I sometimes make gluten-free berry pancakes; the recipe is available on my YouTube channel.) Other excellent whole grains are brown rice, rye, bulgur wheat and quinoa. I also recommend brown pasta and whole-grain, brown sourdough bread.

Limit artificial sweeteners

'Diet' drinks and fizzy drinks have been found to have a negative effect on your gut health.[9] In particular, sweeteners can kill the beneficial bacteria in your gut. As alternatives to artificial sweeteners, I recommend nature's sweetener: fruit. Any fruit that is in season is a great addition to your diet. What about the winter months? During mid-summer, when there is an abundance of fruit on your berry bushes, freeze them so you can have your own, chemical-free berries all winter.

Incorporate more prebiotics in your diet

Prebiotics are a type of fibre that is in a form humans cannot digest. Your gut bacteria feed on this type of fibre, so it naturally increases the amount of gut micro-organisms. You can get supplements that contain prebiotics, but it is better to get them from whole foods for the added advantage of increasing the satiating hormone as you chew. It's also more enjoyable to sit and eat a plate of food than it is to pop a pill. The vegetables listed below are high in a type of prebiotic called inulin (from highest to lowest), which is something your gut microorganisms are mad about:

- Chicory root
- Jerusalem artichoke
- Garlic
- Leeks and onions
- Asparagus

Chicory root

The not-so-commonly found chicory root is a plant related to the common weed, the dandelion. Give it a try. There are also several varieties of salad leaves that are bred from dandelion, including chicory root and endive, typically found in a winter salad bag mix.) Chicory root can also be used in cooking and as a coffee alternative. As chicory root has no caffeine, it has the added benefit of having less of an effect on your sleep.

Jerusalem artichoke

This is quite different from the globe artichoke that you may be familiar with. The Jerusalem artichoke is part of the daisy family, which is obvious if you ever see it flower. Jerusalem artichokes can grow up to 3m tall, but the edible part of the plant is the knobbly tuber, which is rather like a potato. Don't let its appearance put you off. This superfood is not only highly nutritious, but also contains indigestible fibre, which naturally increases your gut micro-organism population. If you decide to grow it yourself, Jerusalem artichoke has other benefits, too. It doesn't get blight, you don't have to earth it up like potatoes and its broad leaves take in large amounts of carbon from the air, helping to reduce global warming. You can eat it raw or grate it into salads, but my favourite recipe is to slice it into strips like crisps, sprinkle them with curry powder and roast them in the oven. It's the new healthy spud.

Garlic

Again, it's the inulin fibre that makes this food so beneficial to your gut health. There is also an antioxidant found in garlic called allicin, which is increased when the garlic clove is chopped and crushed, exposing it to the air. For this reason, my health tip for garlic is to finely chop and crush your cloves before putting them into your stir-fry. Then you can cook it as much as you like. The taste of garlic alone should entice you and it's so easy to add into your diet weekly. If you're worried about smelling of garlic, try baking garlic in olive oil: you'll get all the taste and none of the smell.

Leeks and onions

Leeks and onions are two massively underrated superfoods and should be added to your diet for their flavours alone. Leeks and onions are from the same plant family (alliums) and have similar health benefits, although leeks have a higher inulin content than onions. Leeks are something we don't typically eat enough of. Leeks can be used to make traditional Irish stew, but they can also be used in stir-fries and organic bone broths, which not only improve your gut lining, but also provide you with collagen (contained in the marrow of the bones), which is brilliant for skin health. One of my favourite plant-based dishes is pasta and tofu in creamy leek sauce. (My mouth waters at the thought of it.) This dish has it all. Tofu is a complete protein with all nine essential amino acids. Leeks and garlic are high in fibre (inulin), which your micro-organisms feed on to increase their population. Improved gut health leads to increased production of serotonin in the body. This dish also has complex carbohydrates in the form of organic pasta. These complex carbs give you a slow release of energy, preventing an insulin spike and reducing the number of cravings you have throughout the day. (There is a full video tutorial on my YouTube channel.) If you want to maximise the benefits of onions, eat red onions rather than white. Not only do red onions have more taste, but they also have more antioxidants. (As a general rule, the darker the colour of a vegetable, the higher the antioxidant content.)

There is very little work to growing leeks and onions. For onions, just buy bulbs and plant them into firm ground so that they can get a good hold in the soil, and in four to five months you have a crop. Leeks are slightly different and you get more bang for your buck when you sow them as they are bigger. Sow leeks from seed and transplant out. As the plant grows taller, you should blanch the shanks of the edible stem. (Blanching is the term used for pushing soil up against the stems so that the vegetable develops white stems; it also keeps weeds under control.)

Asparagus

Asparagus also contains inulin – 100 grams (seven medium spears) has 2-3 grams of inulin fibre – but also antioxidants and some plant protein. There are several types of asparagus, including standard green, white and purple. In general, the darker the colour, the higher the antioxidant content, so if purple asparagus is on the menu, you should order that. The antioxidants in purple asparagus are the same as those found in berries and red wine. These antioxidants improve brain function and reduce the signs of ageing without the negative effects of wine such as poor sleep and hangovers.

TOP TIP

As a general rule, the shape and colour of a food item indicates its benefits to particular areas of the body. For example, walnuts resemble tiny brains and contain healthy fats, which improve concentration and brain function.

Carrots, when chopped in rings, look like eyes and contain beta-carotene which makes vitamin A, which improves vision. Beetroot, which is red, is good for your heart as it contains non-heme iron, which improves blood flow. And the shape of asparagus might suggest a certain part of the male anatomy. According to a Chinese proverb, asparagus has the ability to improve erections in men – a proverb that has science to back it up, as asparagus has iron and nitric oxide, which increases blood flow...

Incorporate probiotics in your diet

Probiotics are slightly different from prebiotics in that they contain living good bacteria. These beneficial bacteria can be found in yoghurt and cheese – two of my favourite foods. I don't mean the sugar-sweetened ones with so-called 'natural' flavourings or 'low fat', because the fats found in yoghurt are beneficial to your gut. Eat natural, high-protein yoghurts and add the natural sweetness of fruit. Awareness of probiotics seems relatively recent, given the range of probiotic drinks, supplements and foods on the market today, but knowledge of their beneficial effects has been around for thousands of years. (I don't know if they knew the science behind it or if they just had a good gut feeling. Pun intended!) German sauerkraut and Korean kimchi are both made by fermenting the traditional vegetable, cabbage. The table below lists the fermented foods containing probiotics that I recommend.

All these fermented foods can made at home. The process isn't entirely straightforward, as I discovered (I did not fully submerge the cabbage in its liquid and ended up with a kimchi-flavoured pot handle), but I have now perfected the recipe and method with the use of a kettle bell (see the video on my YouTube channel www.youtube.com/watch?v=0xS8RTkBp0Y).

Kefir	Like yoghurt, this fermented dairy product is a combination of milk and fermented kefir grains, tangy to taste
Kimchi	A traditional Japanese dish related to sauerkraut – fermented cabbage with spices, garlic and carrots
Kombucha (tea)	A fermented, lightly effervescent, sweetened black or green tea
Miso	Fermented soya beans with salt and sometimes rice, barley and seaweed
Natto	A cheesy, stringy, small ball-shaped Japanese dish made from fermented soya beans
Probiotic yoghurt	Fermented milk with added live good bacteria and no added sugars
Raw cheese	Cheese made from fermented, unpasteurised milk (because cooking at high temperatures can kill some beneficial bacteria)
Sauerkraut	Finely shredded cabbage typically fermented in salt water and sometimes berries, making it sour
Tempeh	Fermented soya, high in plant protein, contains non-heme iron

Is it possible to have too much of a good thing in terms of probiotics? The answer is yes. All fermented foods contain histamines, which means that they can cause similar symptoms to mild asthma, such as wheezing and being unable to take deep breaths. When starting my fitness journey, I incorporated fermented foods into every meal. I had an apple cider vinegar shot in the morning (which doesn't help to burn fat, by the way), sauerkraut with lunch, and curry tempeh for dinner, washed down with a kombucha and a yoghurt before bed. Everything was going fine and I was feeling great, except that I was short of breath. Being so in tune with my body, I was able to figure out that the amount of fermented food in my diet needed to be reduced.

Eat organic produce

There has been a huge increase in the number of people suffering from gut issues in recent years, and it's still on the rise. One of the reasons for this is the use of glyphosate, the active ingredient in weedkiller. Typically used in commercial vegetable production, glyphosate is ending up in ever larger amounts in the foods we eat. Glyphosate can damage the lining of your gut. This leads to undigested food particles, bacteria and toxins leaking into the bloodstream and results in inflammation and bloating, so if you eat the skin of fruits or vegetables, make sure they are organic. (See The Clean 15™ and the Dirty Dozen™ in Chapter 5.) If you cannot get an organic fruit or vegetables, then growing them yourself is an option. Failing that, make sure you remove any toxins before you cook or eat them (see 'Removing toxins from vegetables' in Chapter 4).

Gluten intolerance or glyphosate intolerance?

There is also an increasing number of people presenting with poor gut health and being diagnosed with gluten intolerance or celiac disease (not being able to tolerate a husk on wheat). Many people believe that they are gluten intolerant because they become bloated, nauseous or sick when they eat food containing wheat (usually bread). Wheat is one of the world's staple foods and is often offered as a sign of peace (no wonder brown bread is the first thing my granny offers when I bring a potential long-term girlfriend to the house!), but it is often sprayed with weedkillers containing the chemical glyphosate.

Glyphosate has negative effects on your good gut bacteria, leading to nausea, skin rashes, diarrhoea and depression, so before you convince yourself that you are gluten intolerant, try removing non-organic food items from your diet. I am not suggesting that everyone who has been told they have gluten intolerance does not actually have it. Rather, that they might in fact be intolerant of glyphosate. One way to check whether you really are gluten-intolerant or not is to make your own bread. Combine 300 grams organic, gluten-free oats, 500 grams yoghurt, 50 grams pumpkin seeds and an egg in bowl and bake in the oven at 180°C until golden brown.

Feed your gut for improved mood

Have you ever had a 'gut feeling' or 'butterflies' in your stomach? This is due to your stomach sending signals to your brain via your nervous system – specifically, the vagus nerve. This is known as the gut-brain axis. There are more gut micro-organisms in your body than human cells. These micro-organisms can affect your mood, nutritional absorption, weight gain (or loss) and even your brain function. The old adage 'You are what you eat' could not be truer.

There is a daily battle going on in your gut between good and bad bacteria and who wins the war is of huge importance to you. The foods you eat throughout the day will determine whether you have an over-abundance of good or bad gut bacteria. A surfeit of the bad guys can lead to symptoms such as depression, anxiety and obsessive compulsive disorder (OCD). In contrast, an increase in the good bacteria can make us feel relaxed and have a sense of wellbeing (increased serotonin) by releasing GABA (a natural chemical that improves mood).

An ever-increasing number of people are taking anti-biotics (which kill both good and bad bacteria in your gut) as well as anti-depressants (which don't get to the root of problems as they only treat the symptoms). A poor diet of processed foods fortified with vitamins and artificial sweeteners also has negative effects on your gut health. Food is medicine, and cleaning up your diet with high prebiotics, organic foods (any that you can get your hands on) and probiotics could be the secret to unlocking a happier, healthier version of you.

Summary

If you are looking for an improvement in your health, start with your gut. Gut health has a crucial role in your health by helping with digestion, brain function, energy, weight loss, skin health and mood. The best way to improve your gut health is to add natural pre- and probiotic foods to your diet and the best diet is one that consists of local, fresh foods that are organically grown or chemical-free. Toxic chemicals in food, no matter how small the amounts, can cause problems – either now or later in life.

4
Earth And Fibre

As we saw in the previous chapter, there are millions of micro-organisms in our gut, but there are micro-organisms (bacteria and fungi) in the soil, too. These micro-organisms can be seen as a cobweb-like structure under a pile of leaves, for example, which is the joining together of tiny organisms that use the leaf mould as food over winter. Their job is to break down this material to make more nutrients available in the soil.

'Conventional' farmers typically use synthetic, pelleted fertilisers, whereas organic growers use this living material – leaf mould, farmyard manure, grass cuttings – to fertilise the soil in which they grow their crops. To boost the regenerative effect of these natural fertilisers, organic growers use a practice known as 'no dig'. No dig means that the soil is not ploughed, rotavated or dug up.

When I first heard about this, I found it difficult to understand. It works like this: If you don't dig, plough or rotavate the soil, there is minimal disturbance from planting, weeding and harvesting, so you are letting the soil micro-organisms join up and do their job. When the root of a plant attaches to the soil micro-organisms, the root zone is extended and a symbiotic relationship is created.

Other advantages of the no dig system are that it is less labour-intensive (there is no major digging involved), it puts carbon back into the soil (slowing down global warming) and it increases the amount of nutrients in the soil. The no dig system is not only better for the soil, but also better for us, as more vitamins and minerals are absorbed with a larger root zone, so the food is more nutritious.

Nutrients and soil

There is a lot of talk about nutrient-dense foods and the importance of iron, magnesium, calcium and other vitamins, but if the level of these vitamins in the soil is low, they cannot be found in high amounts in fruit, vegetables or other crops grown in that soil. The food we eat today is of less nutritional quality than in previous times because of the state our soil.[10] Over the past fifty years, there has been a dramatic change in the way fruits and vegetables are grown.

A lot of this is due to consumer demand. For example, soft fruits such strawberries, blackberries, raspberries and tomatoes are expected to be available all year round, despite the fact that they are in only season during the warmer summer months. We import them from warmer countries (causing air pollution, which has a negative effect on soil health) and with consumer demand for cheap food from supermarkets, farmers and growers have also been growing higher-yielding crops, which doesn't necessarily mean a higher take-up of nutrients. In doing so, they have selectively bred characteristics such as pest resistance and flavour out of our food. Fruits produced out of season – 'forced fruit' – must be grown hydroponically, in woolly insulation with a drip-feed of nutrients. Flavour and other benefits are sacrificed in this process.

Flavour is linked with antioxidants, which are associated with increased health benefits. When you eat any fresh, in-season organic fruit, whether it be strawberries, tomatoes (technically a fruit) or apples, the taste (not to mention the health benefits) is incomparable with the forced fruit you typically get from the supermarket, which has been harvested while unripe so the flavour has not been able to develop. Even organic fruit or vegetables will not be as beneficial if they are harvested unripe or shipped in from other countries. It's always best to shop locally for your organic food.

You will not only be supporting local business, but also doing something beneficial for the environment, especially if the grower is using regenerative methods to fertilise the soil. In the end, you can't beat Mother Nature's seasonal production process, so aim to eat fruits and vegetables when they're in season in your region. If you can grow your own fruit, do. Plant an apple tree or fruit bush in your garden. You can't get fresher than fruit from your own back yard.

TOP TIP

Harvest soft fruit at peak ripeness and freeze it so that you can have some berries with your porridge on a day where you need to be reminded of sweet summer. Apples have a longer shelf life than soft fruits, so if you have your own apple tree, you can store apples to be stewed. I highly recommend stewing apples with cloves, cinnamon and natural probiotic yoghurt for a healthy alternative to the sugar-laden treats we are accustomed to.

Chemicals

One point that is commonly overlooked is the over-consumption of toxic chemicals in the non-organic foods we eat. Glyphosate is one of the most harmful chemicals and is the main active ingredient in weedkiller. It also speeds up harvesting and therefore reduces costs. Wheat and sugar cane are two common food crops that have high levels of glyphosate sprayed onto them. These foods are typically found in processed breakfast cereals, which are all too common in a standard diet.

While it is generally recommended to eat more fruit and veg, it is also important to eat chemical-free. Some people may argue that tolerably small amounts of chemicals are used in commercial fruit and vegetable production, but I have seen fields sprayed with glyphosate (Roundup) to clear the grass for the next crop. If a herd of beef cattle is then allowed to graze on the sprayed field, then toxic chemicals are found in our food system – both in the animal and in the next veg crop. When soil is sprayed, it doesn't just kill the grass and plants, it also kills soil life and micro-organisms. Without soil micro-organisms, nothing will grow.

If you're looking to reduce the consumption of not only sugar, but also toxic chemicals, you should certainly give processed cereals a skip, no matter how tempting the box may be with its brightly coloured cartoon characters. I'm a big believer in organic overnight oats first thing in the morning – breakfast like a king!

How to remove toxins from vegetables

We have established that toxic chemicals used in the conventional production of fruit and veg can cause negative effects on your gut health, so what steps can you take to remove them? The best way to avoid harsh chemicals is to buy produce labelled 'organic' or 'chemical-free' from a local grower. Organic crops are grown without the use of synthetic fertilisers or pesticides. Quite apart from avoiding toxins, by buying organic (or growing your own) you will also taste the difference, get more nutrients and save yourself money in the long run.

If you do buy commercial fruit and veg, at least wash and scrub them with warm water before you use them as a way to remove some pesticides. Better still, mix two spoonfuls of baking soda with two cups of water and soak the vegetable or fruit for two minutes or more. (The longer you soak it, the more toxins you remove.) Rinse with water before cooking or eating. The longer pesticides sit on fruits and vegetables, the more they are absorbed, so wash your fruit and veg as soon as you get home. In the case of apples, the skin can be peeled to remove the toxins, but when you peel the skin of an apple, you take away the most beneficial part. Most of the antioxidants are found either in the skin, or just below it, and fibre is also in the skin. These nutritional benefits of the skin apply to all fruit and vegetables, so the next time you're peeling carrots before you chop them for cooking, ask yourself, 'Could I just wash the carrots and get the added advantage of higher antioxidants?'

Fibre – what is it?

Fibre is an undigestible carbohydrate (another reason to eat carbohydrates) that makes up all fruits and vegetables and is found in various amounts in different produce. Fibre comes exclusively from plants and there is little or no fibre in meats.

We know that fibre is good for us, but why? High-fibre foods are not typically broken down in the small intestine because fibre is an undigestible carbohydrate. Micro-organisms to the rescue. When these beneficial bacteria in the large intestine (colon) break down the fibre into useable energy, it makes you feel full. When you feel full, you are less likely to have cravings for processed food. (Craving processed foods is never a good thing, no matter how much you try to convince yourself otherwise.) Adding more veg to your diet helps control blood sugar levels, which also prevents cravings, as well as energy highs and lows. Say goodbye to the 3pm slump.

Fibre also helps with the rarely discussed, but common complaint: constipation. Fibre helps move things along, so to speak. When you switch your food choices to curry kale chips instead of fried chips, this will lead not only to weight loss, but to improved gut health as well. High-fibre foods not only keep us fuller for longer, but they also latch on to toxins in the body as they pass through the gut. If left in place, these toxins could build up over time and cause chronic illness such as cancer.

The two main fibres

Fibres are categorised into two main types: soluble and insoluble. Most whole foods contain both types, but typically one is present in larger quantities than the other. It's a balancing act, like anything involved in being fit and healthy.

1. **Soluble fibre:** Soluble fibre slows down digestion by absorbing water from the food to form a gel-like substance in the digestive system. Soluble fibre is found in such foods as (black) beans, broccoli, carrots, peas, nuts, apples, pears, oats and bran. It is also found in fruits and vegetables such as blackberries, raspberries and carrots. Soluble fibre keeps you feeling fuller for longer, thereby reducing cravings. It can even influence your mood.

2. **Insoluble fibre**: Insoluble fibre speeds up the digestion of food by adding substance to your stool, helping to prevent constipation. Foods high in insoluble fibre include wholegrain brown rice, bulgur wheat, quinoa and all vegetables, but especially carrots, parsnips, cauliflower, cucumbers and courgettes. You will see that carrots are included in the lists of both soluble

and insoluble fibre-rich foods. In fact, most fruits and veg have both types of fibre in them.

I'm often asked, 'Which are better for you: fruit or veg?', which is rather like asking, 'Which is your favourite child?', but as a general rule I would say that vegetables typically have more benefits in terms of gut health, as well as having a slight advantage over fruits by containing less natural sugar, which can excessively raise your blood sugar levels.

High-fibre fruits and vegetables

We all know the advice to eat 'five (fruits or vegetables) a day', but how much should be eaten? To get the optimum benefit from fibre, you should aim for a minimum of 21 grams and work your way up to 30 grams of fibre per day. Below is a list of common fruits and veg and the amount of fibre contained in an average 'portion':

To bump up your total fibre intake, simply choose the higher-ranking foods in preference to lower-ranking ones, eg, a pear instead of an apple. (If you haven't tasted an organic pear, you're in for a treat.) What is important – and rarely mentioned – is that it is not merely a question of eating more fibre, but of having a diversity of fibres for a diversity of beneficial gut bacteria. In general, the more diverse the micro-organism population in your gut, the healthier you are.

Vegetables	Fibre	Fruits	Fibre
Black beans (cooked, 100 g)	8.3 g	Avocado (half a medium size, 110 g)	6.8 g
Red kidney beans (cooked, 100 g)	7.4 g	Raspberries (100 g)	6.5 g
Chickpeas (cooked, 100 g)	5.0 g	Blackberries (100 g)	6.4 g
Lentils (cooked, 100 g)	4.6 g	Pear (medium size, 175 g)	5.4 g
Kale (cooked, 100 g)	4.0 g	Apple (medium size, 170 g)	4.2 g
Butternut squash (cooked, 100 g)	3.2 g	Mango (medium size, 200 g)	3.3 g
Carrots (cooked, 100 g)	3.0 g	Banana (medium size, 118 g)	3.1 g
Brussels sprouts (cooked, 100 g)	2.6 g	Orange (medium size, 145 g)	3.5 g
Broccoli (cooked, 100 g)	2.5 g	Grapefruit (medium size, 145 g)	3.4 g
Beetroot (cooked, 100 g)	2.5 g	Banana (medium size, 118 g)	3.1 g
Leeks (cooked, 100 g)	2.0 g	Kiwi (large, 100 g)	3.0 g
Onions (cooked, 100 g)	1.6 g	Blueberries (100 g)	2.4g
Spring onions (100 g)	1.5 g	Tomato (medium size, 100 g)	1.2 g

To achieve this, aim to have twenty to thirty different types of fruits and veg in a week. A recommendation I often give clients is to go to the country market and buy a vegetable that you don't recognise and find a recipe for it. For example, Romanesco (related to broccoli) is a vegetable that is grown in Ireland. I encourage you to get your hands on it. This vegetable not only has fibre, but also contains sulforaphane (a highly-rated antioxidant that binds to free radicals in the body and neutralises them). This antioxidant is also found in broccoli, kale, the humble cabbage and Brussels sprouts. Brussels sprouts are clearly not just for Christmas (they come into season from October).

Don't worry too much about the figures; just eat a wide range of fruits and veg – organic, of course, especially if you are eating the skin. The long and short of it is to choose whole foods as often as possible. The more processed a food item is, the less fibre it typically has. Foods that are less processed typically have a host of vitamins, minerals and antioxidants, which will not only improve your gut health and mood, but also have your body running more effectively from the inside out.

Adding fibre to your diet

Here are some simple tips for increasing your daily fibre intake:

- Add fruit or veg to your breakfast (eg, courgette with oats).
- Have potato wedges with the skins on.

- Roast whole beetroot and eat the skin.

- Swap meat for beans in some meals or add beans to animal products.

- Chop up leeks to include in your stir-fry.

All of these simple hacks can help you to reach your daily fibre intake. Doing this will feed your gut micro-organisms, which will further break down the whole foods you eat, releasing even more nutrients that you can absorb. As a result, you'll have more vitamins and minerals in your body so you can function better with more energy. While it's true that you are what you eat, it is probably more accurate to say, 'You are what you absorb.' With added vitamins and minerals from foods consumed, the body can improve its everyday functions and processes, including cognitive function, healing wounds, bolstering your immune system and promoting normal growth and development of skin, hair and muscle tissue.

When we eat more high-fibre foods, we gain not only benefits from the inside; we feel better on the outside too. This is seen in increased positivity, naturally glowing skin and enhanced energy levels due to our good gut bacteria: micro-organisms. By increasing our fibre intake with a range of different fruits and vegetables, we can naturally populate the gut with a diverse population of gut biome. Having a satisfied and happy gut biome will send positive feedback to the brain, with a direct result that we feel happy and pass on positive vibes.

I don't want you to feel that you cannot enjoy a traditional dish from your country which may have an animal substance in it. My aim is for you to understand what different foods do to your body before you choose a diet that works for you. I'm certainly not advocating adopting a completely meatless diet, but rather to increase the diversity of fruit and veg in your diet so that you can increase the population of micro-organisms in your gut. It pays to add plant-based protein that has fibre, too.

Too much fibre?

A final word of warning: It is possible to have too much fibre in your diet, especially if you go from having very little to eating onions, garlic, beans and greens all in one meal. This can lead to bloating and increased gas because the sudden abundance of fibre increases the number of micro-organisms breaking down that indigestible matter and causes wind. When this occurs, some people say, 'Whole vegetables don't suit me.' The answer is to build up your fibre slowly and space out your vegetable intake throughout the day and week, especially in the case of high-inulin foods from the list above. Oh, and be sure to chew your food.

Summary

Eating fresh food gives you a sense of joy for two main reasons: the extra antioxidants reduce stress on your body and the living micro-organisms found on the skin of vegetables improve the health of your gut. Growing your own gives you a third reason for joy: an improved mood from harvesting a successful crop. In Part Two, I'll be showing you, among other things, how simple it can be to grow your own fruit and veg.

PART TWO
FOOD FOR FITNESS

If there is one thing I love, it's food. If there's something I love even more, it's maximising its benefits. Food is the key thing to focus on if you want to improve your overall health. Sometimes we struggle to know what a healthy food choice is, so in this part of the book I'll be going into some detail on the different kinds of foods and their relative health benefits. As a general rule, I recommend using single-ingredient foods, and when making any meal I start with the vegetables, as let's face it, most of us don't eat enough of them. That's also why I look at vegetables first. Organic food, the gold standard, can sometimes be difficult to source, so I'll be giving you a few pointers on overcoming that challenge in this part of the book too. First though, I want to address the vexing question of 'conventional versus organic'. What are the issues and why should you switch to organic?

5
Conventional Versus Organic

It can be hard to compare the nutritional differences between organic and conventionally grown foods for several reasons. Because different farming methods are used, the crops or vegetables produced are often not comparable. With organic, there is a high standard to be kept with yearly inspections, but with conventional farming, there can be huge variations in methods (some farmers treat land in a similar way to organic methods and others, not so much, eg, grazing animals on land that has just been sprayed). The harvesting method and how long the crop sits in storage before the consumer eats it also affects its nutritional quality. Soil also plays a big part in the nutritional quality of a crop, so what is in the soil – both the good and bad – must also be taken into account (see Chapter 4).

What are the differences?

Soil is the most important living thing in the world. It filters water, it provides nutrients to crops and it prevents global warming. The main difference between conventional and organic farming has to do with the way soil is treated. We have already considered 'no dig' practices in organic farming, but the most significant malpractice of conventional farming is its over-reliance on chemicals: pesticides, herbicides and synthetic fertilisers (see below). These are often made from petrol, and while they do give the soil nutrients, they have a long-term negative effect on the soil, and on the life of every living thing on this planet. The overuse of pesticides and petroleum-based fertilisers is introducing 'invisible toxins' into our fruits and vegetables, including antibiotic drugs and bulking agents.

Certified organic growers, on the other hand, must use regenerative methods of fertilising and controlling and preventing pests and diseases, such as farmyard manure application and stinging nettle, seaweed, comfrey and garlic fertilisers (which also have immune-boosting properties). Organic farming does not rely on chemical intervention to control pests and weeds, but works with the environment to encourage beneficial insects.

Organic growers are more likely to rotate their crops and to grow varieties of fruit and veg that are susceptible to pests and diseases but high in nutrients, even at the cost of lower yields and higher consumer prices. Cheapest is rarely best, and we should be buying produce based on its value to our health rather than its price. Organic animal products are produced without the use of antibiotics, growth hormones or bulking agents. Organically-raised animals are fed organic grain and must be free to roam on seasonal pasture that allows them access to fresh nutrients. In 'exchange', the animals fertilise the fields. Certain kinds of animals (eg, Dexter cattle – a miniature cow) are bred for low compaction of the soil.

Organic certification

For a farm to call itself 'organic', it must be registered with a government body such as the Organic Trust, Irish Organic Association or the Soil Association and then comply with certain standards as set by the EU or the country it is in.

In January 2012, the EU created a Euro Leaf logo for all organic produce. There is a list of countries that have been approved as satisfying the requirements for the use of this green leaf logo found on the official EU website.[11] (Food and feed certified as organic in Great Britain will continue to be accepted as organic in the EU until 31 December 2023.)

To supply certified organic food and have the right to use this logo, a produce must, by law, go through a conversion period of two years. The logo is mandatory for all pre-packaged organic goods and voluntary for non-pre-packaged organic food items. It indicates that the product has complied with the appropriate EU rules and regulations. In the case of processed products such as sauces and creams, the symbol indicates that 95% of the product and its ingredients are registered as organic, with further conditions on the remaining 5%.

In America, the United States Department of Agriculture (USDA) has established its own organic certification logo and processes. Similar strict rules and regulations must be adhered to in order for a product to earn the 'USDA Organic' logo.

Fertilisers, pesticides and weedkillers

Fertilisers

There are two main types of fertilisers typically used to increase crop yield: chemical fertilisers and natural fertilisers. Chemical fertilisers supply nutrients to the soil and are more easily washed out of it (ammonium nitrate, superphosphate and potassium). Natural fertilisers can be found in the form of seaweed, manure (chicken, pig, cattle, horse) and homemade recipes, including garlic, stinging nettle and banana skin (a favourite of mine). Natural fertilisers are more commonly used on smaller organic holdings, where the nutrients take slightly longer to break down and are less likely to run off into our waters.

Pesticides

Pesticides (or insecticides) are chemicals that are used to kill pests, but do so at a cost. They kill both good and 'bad' insects as well as soil micro-organisms and worms. It is now known that pests and insects (unlike humans) can build up a tolerance to pesticides, which means that the chemicals in pesticides end up being more toxic to animals and humans than to the pests themselves. Excessive exposure to pesticides such as glyphosate (the active ingredient found in the world's most widely sold weed killer) affects your endocrine system, which can lead to infertility and cancer.[12]

Pesticides can be applied once, twice or even up to ten times in one growing season. Apples, in particular, are heavily sprayed, making it an easy decision to choose fresh, local organic apples, which become available from September. Closely linked to pesticides are herbicides, fungicides and disinfectants. These all prevent a plant from naturally producing antioxidants, which are linked not only to health benefits, but also with flavour.

Weedkillers

Conventional farming uses a weed killer called Roundup, which contains the active ingredient glyphosate, an antibiotic. One application of Roundup can kill up to 50% of the worm population.[13] Worms are like bees: if they die, so will we. Worms break down soil material into forms that plants can use. Roundup (or a form of it) also acts as an antibiotic, killing both good and bad bacteria in our gut. Remember all the beneficial properties of a healthy gut (see Chapter 4)?

Why is Roundup used if we know how devastating it is? Roundup not only kills weeds, it also speeds up the harvest of some crops, including potatoes, soya and wheat. Science has now come up with a seed that is genetically modified so it can tolerate being sprayed and survive while weeds are killed off. Farmers are told that this will increase yield, but are often not informed as to what it is doing to the soil. It is essential to consider the long-term effects of using Roundup.

Weeds have their own benefits, including providing a haven for beneficial insects to live. The ladybug, with its red-coated body and black spots, is often found on the underside of stinging nettles (if they haven't been sprayed off, that is). Ladybugs are beneficial because they eat destructive aphids such as greenfly.

Nettles are commonly considered as weeds, but even they have their uses. (The definition of a weed is a plant in the wrong place!) Young nettles can be used to improve crops. If they are cut and steeped in a bucket of water overnight with some crushed garlic, this makes a natural 'medicine' that can be sprayed on crops to give them a nitrogen boost, encouraging leafy growth and strengthening their immune system. Both nettles and garlic benefit us with iron and vitamin C, strengthening our overall health. They do the same thing with crops. The antioxidant in garlic is called allicin, which, as I mentioned earlier, is brilliant for the immune system. Young nettle shoots are packed full of vitamin C, which is a natural antihistamine and can help hay fever sufferers – another example of nature providing us with exactly what we need, at the exact time we need it. (Growing up in the country I often ate nettle soup, typically in early spring.)

Numerous studies indicate that that organic food is better for your gut microbiome.[14] As we have seen, eating vegetables that have been exposed to pesticides, especially when the skin of the vegetable is consumed, has an impact on gut health (see Chapter 3). Organic growers are strictly prohibited from using glyphosate to control weeds. Copper-based chemicals are permitted and are typically used to prevent blight, but these can cause toxicity in the body. There are alternatives that prevent the use of copper sprays, such as growing blight-resistant varieties and planting earlier varieties of potatoes so that blight is not a problem. As a general rule, the foods that we eat the skin or leaves of are the most important to get organic, because when sprays are applied, these areas are the chemicals' first point of contact.

Genetically Modified Organisms (GMO)

As we have seen, non-organic farmers can and typically do use GMO seeds, as these can withstand chemicals and will produce higher yields. Some people think that GMO is the future because we need more food to feed the world's ever-increasing population, but in the developed world we waste close to a third of the food we produce.[15] We are currently producing too much cheap, low-grade food such as spinach that has been washed in chlorine (the smell hits you the second you open the bag) and turns to mush after a few days.

Given what we have seen of conventional farming methods, we also need to consider the long-term consequences of using harsh chemicals such as glyphosate. As we know, reduced soil health due to excess spraying has negative effects on our gut. I highly recommend that you choose organic foods, especially if you are looking to improve your health in the long term.

Nutritional value

Some studies suggest there is little difference in nutritional value between organic and non-organic foods, particularly in terms of magnesium, iron, and vitamins A, B, D and K.[16] However, with organic food, it is not so much what is in it, as what is *not* in it: harsh chemicals (which have been proven to cause the body to function at less-than-optimal levels) and, in excessive amounts, contribute to gut issues, skin problems and chronic illness.[17] Research also indicates that there is more omega-3 in organic produce than conventional. As we have seen, omega-3 is an essential healthy fat that we need in our diet (see Chapter 2).[18]

Antioxidants

The majority of studies indicate that organic produce has higher levels of antioxidants than conventional produce.[19] Why are these important?

In simple terms, antioxidants are compounds that prevent cell damage. These beneficial chemical compounds are found naturally in various fruits and vegetables. (There are negligible amounts in animal tissue.) Antioxidants are produced in fruits and vegetables and prevent or reduce damage from pests and disease. When we consume whole foods that contain antioxidants, we obtain their beneficial properties.

Antioxidants not only improve the flavour of fruits and vegetables, but also protect our bodies from ageing and reduce stress. They can prevent – and in some cases even reverse – serious illness.[20] When your body is less stressed, you have more energy. When you have more energy, you are much more likely to exercise, and when you exercise, you are more likely to reach your fitness goals. You will also be more productive, which may get you a rise at work (you can thank me later). If you take nothing else from this book, remember that the more antioxidant-rich foods you eat, the better.

Free radicals

To understand antioxidants and their role, we also need to know about free radicals. Essentially, if antioxidants are the good guys, free radicals are the bad guys. Free radicals are toxic particles that we ingest by breathing toxins in the air or consuming chemically produced fruits and vegetables. A build-up of free radicals in the body leads to increased stress, lowers energy levels and prevents the body from functioning at its best. A build-up of free radicals also plays a major role in the development of inflammation – everything from a slight swelling of any part of your body (often your stomach, bloating is a sign) to rashes, acne and more chronic diseases such as cancer.

Antioxidants neutralise free radicals, help to speed up muscle recovery, reduce inflammation, slow the skin's ageing process and improve skin health. When we ingest foods that contain a high level of antioxidants, they act as a defence mechanism against free radicals.

Antioxidants and food

When food is produced organically and not sprayed with toxic chemicals, there is a significant increase in these tiny, yet powerful micronutrients: antioxidants. Research shows that there are higher amounts of anti-oxidants in organic produce versus conventional.[21] When organic food is growing, it is more likely to be stressed by small insects nibbling on its leaves. A plant can't get up and walk away from a stressful situation as we can, so it produces antioxidants. These act as its first line of natural defence. For example, a tomato plant may be attacked by bugs biting its leaves, which we typically don't eat. In response, the tomato plant produces antioxidants, which end up in the fruit.

Another benefit of antioxidants is that they are linked with flavour. An organically grown tomato is not only more tolerant to pests attacking it, but it also produces a more delicious fruit. That is one of the reasons why home-grown or organic tomatoes taste so much better.

Organic meats don't have a lot of antioxidants, which is why I recommend getting more fruit and veg into your diet. Antioxidants are found in every fruit and vegetable that you can think of. Herbs and spices are extremely high in antioxidants too. Because of this (as well as for flavour), I use them in every meal in my *Organic Fitness Cookbook*.[22] If you do eat organic meat, you will get other benefits: no antibiotics, no growth hormones and higher omega-3 content from the animals being raised on grassland for a high percentage of their life cycle. Antioxidants can also be bought in powdered or tablet form, but it's far better to get them from whole foods, with all their added benefits.

Four main types of antioxidants

There are four main types of antioxidants. The colour of a fruit or vegetable gives an indication of which antioxidant it contains. From this we can determine its potential health benefits:

1. **Red = lycopene:** Lycopene is commonly found in tomatoes, peppers, goji berries, pomegranates, watermelons and grapefruit. It is a powerful antioxidant that protects the skin from sun damage, reduces stress and can help prevent the symptoms of some cancers, including breast and prostate cancer.[23] Lycopene has also been found to improve cholesterol levels, reducing the risk of premature heart disease.[24]

2. **Orange and yellow = beta carotene:** Beta carotene is found in carrots, sweet potatoes and butternut squash. The body converts this antioxidant into vitamin A. Beta carotene is beneficial in improving cognitive function and vision and preventing some cancers.[25] I'm frequently asked if it's better to cook a vegetable or eat it raw. If you're thinking that raw is the better option, you're right. If you think that cooking them is better, you're also right.

For example, carrots increase their antioxidants when cooked, while antioxidant levels in peppers decrease when cooked (especially when oven roasted). I suggest adding peppers into a stir-fry at the last minute to warm them up or eating them raw like an apple.

3. **Purple and blue = anthocyanin:** Anthocyanin is something we typically don't get enough of. This purple antioxidant can reduce the signs of ageing and speed up blood flow, resulting in more energy and reduced wrinkles.[26] Foods that are packed with anthocyanin include red cabbage (which is really purple, not red), blueberries, blackberries and also one of my favourite foods: beetroot. Make sure you add more purple-coloured foods to your diet.

4. **Green = chlorophyll:** The green colour that is found in all dark, leafy greens indicates the presence of chlorophyll. You can incorporate greens into your breakfast by adding spinach to savoury oats, and into lunches and dinners with a salad of chard or salad rocket (arugula) or a kale stir-fry. Most people have heard of chlorophyll and how it makes food for the plant by a process called photosynthesis, but what can it do for us? Chlorophyll not only improves skin health and speeds up wound healing; it can also help stop the development of cold sores with its anti-viral properties.[27] As a known anti-inflammatory, it reduces redness in damaged skin, and if you suffer from acne, greens are one of the first things to add to your diet.[28]

The Dirty Dozen™ and the Clean 15™

Each year, the Environmental Working Group (EWG) updates its list of the twelve foods that are the most heavily sprayed (The Dirty Dozen™) and the fifteen foods that are the least heavily sprayed (the Clean 15™).[29] The EWG compiles this list from US Department of Agriculture data. In 2021, the lists were (in order of 'dirtiest' and 'cleanest' foods):

Dirty Dozen™	Clean 15™
1. Strawberries	1. Avocados
2. Spinach	2. Sweetcorn
3. Kale/Collard/Mustard greens	3. Pineapples
4. Nectarines	4. Onions
5. Apples	5. Papayas
6. Grapes	6. Frozen sweet peas
7. Cherries	7. Eggplant
8. Peaches	8. Asparagus
9. Pears	9. Broccoli
10. Bell and hot peppers	10. Cabbage
11. Celery	11. Kiwi fruit
12. Tomatoes	12. Cauliflower
	13. Mushrooms
	14. Honeydew
	15. Cantaloupe

The foods in the Dirty Dozen™ are the most important foods to consume chemical-free or organic. They are also foods that I recommend growing yourself. You may be surprised not to find broccoli on this list, but its huge, palm-shaped leaves protect the most edible part of the plant from the brunt of the sprays. If you do eat a lot of it, it's still worth getting organic in order to reduce the number of pesticides going into your body.

Summary

The production of non-organic foods can involve the use of harsh chemicals sprayed from top-to-toe not just once, but typically several times in a growing season. Organic meat and produce are not given growth hormones or antibiotics that have negative effects on our gut health. It can be argued that non-organic foods only use small amounts of chemicals, which are well under recommended limits, but the fewer chemicals in your food, the better.

The benefits of organic versus non-organic produce in terms of nutritional value may be subject to debate, but the higher antioxidant levels in organic foods make them a much better choice. Eating organic food is not only beneficial for us, it's also better for the soil, which has a huge part to part to play in future food supply.

In response to the argument that organic food is too expensive, I advise you to grow it yourself. The constant argument of whether organic or conventional food is 'better' can be thrown out of the window when you grow your own. Failing that, you can order organic food from a box scheme that delivers it to your door, which is becoming more popular with the increase in demand. Going to a country market is another option.

If you decide to add one more piece of organic food to your diet or plant just one of the vegetables or fruits I recommend in the following chapters, you will see, taste and feel the benefit. It's easy to incorporate organic food into your diet, with organic salad greens and fruit readily available at most times of the year.

Organic is, of course, the gold standard of food, with its added benefits of higher antioxidant content, but it's important to point out that eating a non-organic strawberry is still by and large a healthier choice than eating junk food.

6
Organic Fitness Foods: Vegetables 1

In the next four chapters I am going to talk about the top organic fitness foods, starting with the most important of all: vegetables. There are so many of these, and they're so important to your health and fitness, that there are two chapters on them, arranged alphabetically. After that come fruits, herbs and spices, and finally, in Chapter 9, meat, dairy products and other foods.

The nutritional value of any fruit or vegetable decreases the second it is harvested. Losses of vitamins occur as the fruit or vegetable is transported, stored on site and left to sit on the shelf of a shop and then in your fridge. This is why I recommend growing your own fruit and veg whenever possible and I will give you planting, cultivating and harvesting tips as well as buying, cooking and eating advice for each food.

When people say they don't like vegetables, what they are often referring to is veg that was harvested two weeks ago, transported halfway across the world and then boiled to within an inch of its life. Fresh vegetables taste completely different.

Asparagus – the 'superfood'

Asparagus is a slightly odd-looking vegetable, but don't let that put you off eating it. Asparagus uniquely finds its way into the top seven natural prebiotics that are good for gut health. As we now know, good gut health is linked with an improved immune system, so you are less likely to fall ill and are healthier overall.

Benefits of asparagus

The benefits of including asparagus in your diet are almost endless. To begin with, asparagus is nutrient-packed: a bunch of five spears contains over 25% of both your daily iron and vitamin A requirements. It also contains vitamin B6, which can improve mood; vitamin C, which is good for cell repair and skin health, resulting in fewer wrinkles; and vitamin K, which is helpful to the body for wound healing and blood clotting. All these benefits for just 20 calories.

Asparagus contains anti-inflammatory properties that help reduce the swelling of any cell. This has a range of effects, from keeping your face and body free of spots to helping prevent chronic illnesses. Including asparagus in your diet can help your body utilise the carbohydrates you consume more effectively, as it contains vitamin B1, which is important for your metabolism. Carbohydrates are important as they are the body's first source of energy, but they are even more beneficial when consumed with foods that contain vitamin B1.

Finally, asparagus has an effect on your hormones. My first encounter with it was on a trip to a country market, where bold letters on a piece of cardboard proclaimed, 'Improve your sex drive with this vegetable!' Being a curious (as well as health-conscious) individual, I was intrigued. Not only did I buy some to try it out for myself, but I was keen to research more about this bold claim. This led me to scientific confirmation that asparagus:

- Improves erectile function in men
- Balances oestrogen and progesterone in women
- Increases libido in both men and women[30]

I have been buying asparagus ever since – from early spring, when it starts to come into season.

Buying, cooking and growing asparagus

When buying asparagus, choose spears that have firm buds and snap when you bend them (probably best to get to ask the grower to do a snap test for you!). When cooking asparagus, to reduce the loss of vitamins and minerals, roast in a low oven, lightly steam them or grate them raw over your meal. Adding in hemp seeds increases your body's absorption of the fat-soluble vitamin A, as well as providing extra protein, omega-3 and magnesium. Hemp seeds are a staple on my Organic Fitness Training Program for that very reason: being a non-meat, complete protein source, containing essential omega-3 healthy fats and being low in carbohydrates.

Asparagus is a plant that comes back year after year. All you have to do is plant a single seed in spring. 'That's my kind of crop,' I hear you say. Quite apart from nutritional value and health benefits, it's a rewarding process to sow a seed and see it develop into a plant. It's recommended that you not harvest any asparagus spears until the plant's third year to allow it to fully establish its root system. To shorten the time until you can harvest your own, you can buy what is called a crown. It looks like an octopus. Just plant the crown in free-draining soil (a raised bed is perfect) and you can harvest your own asparagus from year one with very little work.

Beetroot – better than a banana

The diet that I eat now is in many ways different from what I once ate. Don't get me wrong – we had as healthy meals as any two parents working full-time, twelve-hour shifts as psychiatric nurses could provide, but beetroot was not commonly eaten at our house. Because of its many health benefits, beetroot is now easily one of my favourite vegetables to eat, cook and grow. One of my lecturers (later a mentor of mine) once advised us not to be alarmed about the pinkish-red tinge of our urine after eating a lot of beetroot. (I didn't believe him at the time, but it's true: the pink tinge is due its antioxidants.)

Beetroot belongs to the same family as spinach and chard and comes in yellow, green, white, as well as red varieties. There is even a variety of beetroot called 'bullseye' that has rings of red and white and resembles a dartboard and one that is bright orange (the sweetest). Trying these different types will get varied antioxidants into your diet, but is also a great way into induce kids to eat more veg.

Beetroot is great value, as the whole plant can be eaten. In fact, the long stems are some of the best parts of it. The leaves have a similar taste to kale, and the round root is sweet as the majority of the plant's natural sugars are found there.

Benefits of beetroot

Beetroot has a high nitrate content, which brings great health benefits. Nitrates help improve the body's blood-flow. When more blood is pumped around the body, your muscles work more efficiently from receiving the increased oxygen carried in the blood. When your muscles function more effectively, you have more energy. Increased energy allows you to perform at your best in both your day-to-day tasks and your training (or any exercise, for that matter). It is a no-brainer, then, to add beets to your diet.

The brain is a muscle, too, so beetroot has the same beneficial effects on your brain. A single meal including a nitrate-rich food such as beetroot (or rocket, spinach or parsley) can improve cognitive function, resulting in the ability to think more clearly – food for thought, literally. People who play sports often take beetroot shots before a game – not only to maximise their available energy, but also to speed up their reaction time. Beetroot also has more potassium than a banana. Potassium helps regulate the fluid in your body and prevents muscles from getting weak. It isn't common to see tennis players munching on a beetroot between games, but you never know – the current generation of health nuts could start a new trend... The thing that's missing in a beetroot shot is fibre, so eat the whole veg to maximise the benefits.

The purple colours in beetroot and its leaves contain the antioxidant anthocyanin. Although this can also be found in grapes and berries, vegetables are lower in sugars. As a child, you may have been told to eat your greens, but my advice is to eat your purples.

Buying, cooking and growing beetroot

Beetroot is best eaten cooked. It contains oxalates that reduce the absorption of the iron found in beetroot and cooking removes these oxalates. I suggest cutting beetroot into rings and steaming it as you would potatoes before adding it to your smoothies or as a low-calorie, nutrient-dense side dish.

Beetroot is close to being the perfect crop to grow in your back garden. It is susceptible to very few pests and diseases; even slugs don't seem to bother it. Beetroot seeds come in small clusters that look like miniature grenades. Sow them in small, recycled yoghurt pots to give them a head-start on a warm window sill or glasshouse, or directly into weed-free soil. They should be sown 2cm deep (roughly the depth of the last phalanx on your index finger) and 10cm apart (roughly the width of your fist) in early March. Harvest them eight weeks later for baby beets or twelve weeks for larger ones. Beetroot can be stored in sand over the winter, so eaten all year round.

Brilliant broccoli

When I was growing up, I used to go on 'working holidays' to a relative's farm in Cork. At mealtimes, potatoes and carrots were the typical veg on offer, but occasionally broccoli was served. The family had a son who was a fussy eater. He would only eat the broccoli stems, so I was the lucky winner of extra broccoli heads, but you don't have to have a fussy eater in the house to benefit from more broccoli. Indeed, there's no sense in being fussy with broccoli, because to maximise its benefits (as well as reduce food waste) you should eat the whole plant.

Broccoli is one of the family of brassica vegetables, which includes kale, Brussels sprouts, cauliflower, cabbage, rocket, radish and kohlrabi (German for 'cabbage turnip'). Brassica vegetables are often rejected due to their bitter taste. The distinctive taste, however, is linked to the antioxidants found in them – one of their principal health benefits.

Benefits of broccoli

I call it 'brilliant broccoli' because of its many health benefits. Broccoli contains vitamins C and A, iron, magnesium and fibre, which collectively improve the immune system and skin health, increase energy and improve gut health. There is also a powerful antioxidant found in broccoli (and all other brassica vegetables) called sulforaphane, so if broccoli is out of season or not in stock, reach for its cousins. Sulforaphane, however, becomes deactivated in the cooking process. This reduces its benefits, so it's important to eat broccoli raw if you want to be really healthy. If you're not keen on raw broccoli, some other eating suggestions are given below.

Buying, cooking and growing broccoli

As soon as you get your broccoli heads home, put the 'trunk' in water so that it stays fresh for longer. Broccoli should always be cut to allow air to get to the cells of the plant so that it produces sulforaphane. Exposing the cut pieces to the air for forty minutes will let the antioxidant develop fully. If you can't wait forty minutes, add mustard seeds (which broccoli and other brassicas are grown from) or raw greens such as rocket or mizuna salad leaves to your cooked broccoli, which will reactivate this beneficial compound.

Broccoli is one of my favourite vegetables, not only for its health benefits, but also because of its versatility in cooking. It's preferable to steam it to reduce further losses of other vitamins such as vitamin C. You can use the water from the steamed broccoli in a broth. This idea came to me when I lived in Australia and was learning to cook. I'd steam pretty much all my vegetables to go with what I thought at the time was the one meal you had to eat to be healthy: chicken and broccoli with potatoes or rice. I realised that I could drink the water I'd used to steam the veg instead of pouring it down the sink. (At the time, this was a revelation to me.)

I also used to steam a lot of sweet potatoes, which were common in Australia at the country markets, and I thought I'd come up a new health craze: sweet potato tea! When I rang my dad and excitedly told him about my brilliant new concept, he informed me that he had been doing this for years, so my hope of being fitness famous at twenty-four came crashing down.

You can also roast it with other in-season veg like garlic and onions, using coconut oil to increase the absorption of vitamins A and K. Pan-frying broccoli in stir-fry fashion is my preferred way of cooking it, for two reasons: added crunch (signalling to the brain that you are eating) and less washing-up!

Broccoli stems are often deemed inedible, but if you cut them into small chunks and add them to a stir-fry, they'll be quite tasty and you'll get the best bang for your buck. If you still think the stems are a bit too hard to eat, you can lightly peel them, but remember that most of the benefits of foods are found in the skin or just below it – yet another reason to get organic broccoli heads and eat the whole stem.

When I started growing my own vegetables, broccoli was the crop that I was really looking forward to growing, but I soon learned that it is not the easiest of veg to grow. To begin with, a seed of broccoli in April will produce only one or two heads in three months compared with, for example, salad rocket (arugula), which produces a healthy crop just four weeks later. As I also discovered, a pest called the flea beetle, which thrives in summer, will bite small holes in the leaves of any of the brassica crops, making them look as if they have been attacked with a shotgun. Not only does this make them unsightly, but the crop is also prevented from establishing. Using a type of netting that prevents this pest getting at your plants is a game-changer for anyone growing brassica crops. I use lengths of plastic water pipe bent into hoops to create a mini-polytunnel.

Another challenge of growing broccoli is one of its growing traits. When broccoli starts to produce its head (the edible flower bit), one day it can look nearly ready to pick and the next day be gone too far. This is one reason why most people don't grow their own broccoli on a small scale, but the benefits surely outweigh the tribulations of growing your own.

Carrots of all colours

Carrots have been a part of the Irish diet for centuries. They are easy to grow, they store well, and they can make you see in the dark (or so my granny says!). Carrots were originally dark purple, as they contained that antioxidant anthocyanin (which we typically don't get enough of). The Dutch were the first to selectively breed carrots so that their colour changed from purple to white to yellow and then to the distinctive orange colour we recognise today. You can get also rainbow carrots, which have a multitude of colours. Growing these or purple carrots is well worth a try, not only to entertain kids, but also because of the different antioxidants you'll get from the varied colours.

Mashed carrots are probably one of the first vegetables we eat as babies. In fact, most of us continue to have carrots for the whole of our childhood, for good reasons. You will already know that carrots are good for our sight. Orange vegetables contain the antioxidant beta carotene, which is converted into vitamin A and this causes you skin to become brighter. During my health and fitness journey, I switched to eating carrots (and sweet potatoes), rather than white potatoes with chicken as a protein source. After a number of weeks of consuming these orange-coloured vegetables pretty much every day, however, the palms of my hands started to look as if I'd applied fake tan. This anecdote is not intended to discourage you from eating orange-coloured foods, but to show you the power of foods and their antioxidants on the body. Consuming beta carotene/vitamin A can give your face a healthy glow, which is often said about people who have a lot of veg in their diet. Just make sure not to overdo it – orange palms are not the look we're going for!

The benefits of carrots

Vitamin A is needed for all functions of the cells within the skin and it helps the skin to retain its elasticity. By eating just two small carrots (100 grams), you will exceed your daily vitamin A requirements. With the benefits of better skin health (one of the first signs of a person's overall health), improved vison and immune system, wound healing and the prevention of certain chronic diseases, you would be crazy not to eat carrots. Carrots are often mentioned as a high-carb veg, but if there has ever been a case of someone gaining weight because they ate too many carrots, I've yet to hear about it.

Which are better: carrots or parsnips? Carrots and parsnips are often paired. They are quite similar in nutritional value but differ in their plant families. Like carrots, parsnips are nutritionally solid vegetables to add to your diet and store well in sand for the winter months. Note, however, that when root vegetables are stored in sand, they sometimes send out shoots, as they think that they are in soil and should be growing. Twisting off the shoots that emerge from the tops of the carrots is not a problem, but in the case of parsnips, it can be. Parsnips also belong to the same family as hog weed, whose sap can cause serious burns if it comes into direct contact with the skin. During one of the first growing seasons, I twisted the tops off some parsnips with my bare hands only to end up with blisters. For this reason, I prefer carrots, but also eat parsnips.

Buying, cooking and growing carrots

Purchasing carrots with the dirt still on them is the best way to keep them fresh for longer, as soil is a natural preservative. When I think of carrots, the image of Bugs Bunny biting on a raw carrot comes to mind. If only he knew that he could have increased his absorption of vitamin C if he'd cooked that carrot! Lightly sauteing your carrots makes the cell walls of the edible root crop softer, making it easier for our digestive system to break down the vitamin C and other nutrients. Also, eat them with a healthy fat in order to maximise their benefits, as vitamin A is a fat-soluble vitamin that increases its absorption in the body.

Carrots are sown directly into the ground and there is nothing better than a freshly-pulled carrot from your garden. There is one main problem with growing carrots, however: a pest called the carrot root fly. The carrot root fly has two life cycles, so in order to minimise its effect on my carrot crop, I sow my carrots in late May and cover them with netting. (If you rustle the foliage of the carrots, this gives off the lovely smell of sweet carrots, which attracts the carrot root fly to your crop, so resist the temptation!) Apart from pest prevention and the occasional weeding, carrots are a low-maintenance, nearly fool-proof crop.

If growing on a small scale, it's best to sow them 1cm deep in drills 25cm (about the length of your foot) apart, with 4cm (the length of the end of your thumb) between seeds. Carrots will germinate in about two weeks. We have talked about the millions of micro-organisms found in our gut, and some of these can be found on carrots, so when you harvest a fresh carrot, lightly dust off the soil and take a bite.

French beans

French beans, also known as green beans, are an affordable, sustainable protein source that vegans and vegetarians typically eat.

Benefits of French beans

If there are two main things that people don't get enough of in their diets, it's protein and fibre, and French beans are a great source of both. French beans are not a complete protein source on their own, but they can be paired with other foods that have the missing links to make a complete protein: nuts, seeds, grains, eggs, cheese, fish or meat if you eat them. French beans can be eaten raw, straight off the plant or in a salad. I enjoy a combination of rocket greens, spring onions, French beans, steamed beetroot and fresh tomatoes cut cold onto the plate. I also add a protein source such as hemp seeds. (They'll bump up your heathy fats and fibre, too.) Spice it all with pink salt. French beans are not only a protein source, but also a source of vitamin C, which people often down a daily vitamin C tablet for.

Buying, cooking and growing French beans

You can, of course, buy tinned beans, but fresh ones have beneficial, living micro-organisms on them – and the sooner you get them from farm to fork, the better. French beans also supply the soil with nitrogen, which is needed for growth, so French beans are well worth growing as well as adding to your diet.

French beans grow better inside in warmer conditions, so a glasshouse or polytunnel is ideal. Train them up a trellis or along a string line. Plant 2cm deep and 30cm apart. I recommend the Cobra variety for a high yield. Fifteen seeds are sufficient for a manageable bean crop for a typical family. A final growing tip: The more you pick, the more beans the plant will produce. If you leave the beans unharvested, the plant will use its energy to produce seeds rather than making more delicious beans.

7
Organic Fitness Foods: Vegetables 2

In this chapter I continue my A-Z (well, A-Y actually) of organic vegetables: why they're good for you and how to buy, cook and grow them.

Jerusalem artichokes (nothing like globe artichokes)

This is not the first time I've mentioned Jerusalem artichokes (see Chapter 3 on gut health). Jerusalem artichokes are completely different from globe artichokes. The main difference is that the edible part of the globe artichoke grows above the ground, whereas the edible part of the Jerusalem artichoke grows below the soil like a potato.

The benefits of Jerusalem artichokes

Jerusalem artichokes are beneficial to your diet because they contain a specific type of fibre: inulin. This vegetable and its effects are so strong that you will start to feel the effect on your gut within ten minutes. It is important to introduce Jerusalem artichokes into your diet gradually – they are also known as fart-a-chokes! The passing of wind, though, is a natural process and a sign that your gut microbes are working.

Buying, cooking and growing Jerusalem artichokes

When buying Jerusalem artichokes, pick out the darker (purple) ones and go with the smoother variety, as this makes them easier to wash. Jerusalem artichokes are carbohydrates and can be steamed or roasted like potatoes, grated onto salads and eaten raw or sliced into strips like crisps, sprinkled with curry powder and roasted in the oven.

As for growing your own, Jerusalem artichokes, like potatoes, are edible tubers. All you have to do is stick them in the ground. They involve little or no weeding, attract bees and take in carbon from the air, doing their bit to slow down global warming. Even if you don't have a current veg patch, you can create one as you plant your Jerusalem artichokes. Get some old farmyard manure or seaweed and spread it on the ground (or grass) over an area 2m long and

1m wide. Next, turn the grass sod and soil into the seaweed or manure, making ridges the width of the shovel. (Incidentally, this is great exercise.) Plant your Jerusalem artichokes into the ridges, using the topsoil from the trench to cover the tubers. You can also use this planting technique with garlic cloves. Plant the tubers in February and you can harvest them at the tail-end of the same year (when nature intended us to eat them) to improve your immune system going into winter.

Kale – magnesium-rich

Kale, a member of the brassica family like broccoli, not only has antioxidants like sulforaphane, but also contains magnesium, which is frequently lacking in our diets. Kale comes in a variety of colours, including green and purple, both of which I urge you to incorporate into your diet.

Benefits of kale

Magnesium is used in over 300 different processes in the body. It helps to maintain normal nerve and muscle function, supports a healthy immune system and keeps the heartbeat steady. It also helps increase energy levels by aiding in regulating levels of glucose, which is converted from the carbohydrates we eat. Due to its role in our nerve functioning, magnesium also helps reduce anxiety. Most dietary magnesium comes from dark green, leafy vegetables.

The high magnesium content in kale also helps with sleep, not only setting us up for a successful day ahead, but also allowing our body, muscles and skin to recover. Kale is also a good source of vitamins C and A. These vitamins are easily absorbed and also help improve skin.

TOP TIP

Magnesium is typically found in multivitamins and you can even take magnesium tablets, but you miss out on the fibre if you do. Other foods that are good sources of magnesium include:

- Fruits (bananas, dried apricots and avocados)
- Nuts (almonds and cashews)
- Whole grains (brown rice and millet)
- Soy products (tempeh and tofu)
- Peas, beans and seeds (flax seeds, chia seeds and pumpkin seeds)

Buying, cooking and growing kale

When buying kale, don't buy the 'dead stuff' as my sister calls it. Nutrients are lost from a vegetable the second it is harvested, so if it has gone limp it has already lost a good deal of goodness. If your kale starts to go limp when you get it home, put the base of it in water to perk it up again. My favourite way to cook kale is to sprinkle it with curry powder and bake it in the oven for five to ten minutes for delicious curry kale chips.

Kale is one of the hardiest winter vegetables and one of the easiest to grow. The purple kale variety called Midnight Sun grows particularly well. (It even sounds cool!) Another variety, Nero di Toscana (also known as dinosaur kale), is often on 5-star hotel menus; save yourself a whole lot of money by growing it yourself. To grow kale, sow one seed in small trays or pots 2cm deep and then transplant into your garden bed. As the transplant grows, only take the lower leaves and just three plants will have you eating kale for breakfast, lunch and dinner. One final tip is to push soil up around the stem for support, because as you strip the lower leaves, the plant looks a lot like Beaker from *Sesame Street*.

'Magic' mushrooms

No, I'm not referring to *those* magic mushrooms; I'm saying that ordinary mushrooms are magic, too. Mushrooms have been used for thousands of years and there are lots of different types in a variety of sizes, shapes and colours. Mushrooms grow wild, but are more commonly grown in grow room chambers and cultivated.

While mushrooms can be beneficial to our health, some are also extremely poisonous, which is why it is best practice to buy them at a local farmer's market or in store rather than foraging through the woods in search of a side dish for tonight's dinner. The most common mushrooms on the market are:

- Button or white
- Portobello
- Oyster
- Shiitake
- Lion's mane

Benefits of mushrooms

I did not fully appreciate mushrooms until I learned about their benefits. I used to think of them as a whole lot of nothingness. Boy, was I wrong. Mushrooms may be small, but they have big health-boosting benefits. Research shows that they have the ability to boost your immune system, kill off harmful diseases and aid in healthy liver function.[31] While all vegetables have fibre, mushrooms have a type of fibre called beta glucan. Beta glucan is one of the fibres most people lack in their diet. Oyster and shiitake mushrooms are particularly high in beta glucan – another reason I decided to grow them. (It's also found in wholegrain breads, yeast, seaweed and algae.) It's a soluble fibre that slows down bowel movements and prevents sugar spikes, making it a perfect food for controlling diabetes. Anyone suffering with insulin resistance and Type 2 diabetes should consider adding mushrooms to their diet for the main reason of preventing insulin spikes.

Mushrooms are one of the few foods to contain a certain protein called ergothioneine (ET), which is one of the few proteins that can penetrate the mitochondria, the powerhouse of the cell. ET acts as an antioxidant to reduce inflammation and prevent excessive oxidation inside the mitochondria. (Other foods that contain smaller amounts of ET, as well as fibre and plant protein, include black beans and kidney beans.) Last, but not least, mushrooms are a great plant-based source of B vitamins, which are essential for the body to function at optimal levels. Here's a summary of what these B Vitamins do:

- **B2:** Plays an important role in defending your body from free radicals and preventing excessive inflammation and stress.

- **B3:** Aids in breaking down energy from the food we eat. B3 also supports normal nervous system functioning, while improving skin health and preventing fatigue.

- **B5:** Helps your body convert carbohydrates into energy. B5 is also involved in making hormones such as melatonin, which helps improve sleep.

- **B6:** Makes and breaks down protein that we consume. B6 also plays a role in brain health, protecting cells and making hormones such as serotonin (the happy hormone).

Mushrooms are not only packed full of B vitamins, they also contain high levels of vitamin D. Vitamin D, also known as the 'sunshine vitamin', is a natural mood improver. The body can only produce vitamin D when the skin is exposed to direct sunlight. The sun, however, is extremely seasonal-dependent, so mushrooms are particularly important during those long, dark winter months. It's important to note that the amount of vitamin D in mushrooms can vary because they must be exposed to UV light or direct sun to get vitamin D. This illustrates the importance of knowing where and how your food is produced.

Buying, cooking and growing mushrooms

Buy your mushrooms at a shop that gets regular, fresh deliveries and organise your shopping day to match. Mushrooms should look fresh and smell good. Avoid mushrooms that have signs of mildew or mould or wet patches.

The best way to cook mushrooms while preserving their nutritional properties is to grill them, as frying at high temperatures or boiling them reduces their antioxidant activity. Fried mushrooms, in particular, have significantly less protein and carbohydrate content and an increase in fat.[32] They are, of course, also delicious raw – in a salad or dipped in home-made guacamole.

You can get DIY kits for growing a small quantity of mushrooms, which you put in a dark, cool place (eg, under your sink). Shiitake mushrooms stand out for me both for their noted health benefits and also for their ability to grow in freshly cut Alder wood. The timber for the mushrooms to grow in must be freshly cut and seasoned in a cool, dry area for two weeks before the first step of drilling holes in the timber and placing fungi into them, known as the inoculation phase.

Potatoes – the versatile vegetable

Potatoes are a versatile vegetable that is a staple food in many households for a number of reasons. Potatoes are relatively inexpensive, easy to grow and packed full of nutrients.

Benefits of potatoes

Potatoes contain iron, vitamin C and potassium. Iron is commonly deficient in our diets, particularly in women due to their menstruation cycles. Vitamin C helps speed up the recovery of your skin or muscle cells and potassium helps regulate the fluid in your body and prevents muscles from getting weak.

100g or a medium-sized potato has a similar amount of potassium to a banana. This is why bananas are a good snack to have just before training. Unlike potatoes, however, bananas aren't easily grown in Ireland – or the rest of Europe or most of America, for that matter.

There are so many different varieties of potato. Pink Fir is a silky-smooth potato with a finger and knuckle shape. Arran Victory is a purple-skinned potato that – you guessed it – has more antioxidants than the regular ones we typically eat. The antioxidants are nearly all found in the skin of the potato, which I encourage you to eat. Another antioxidant-rich potato is Violetta, which is purple the whole way through. I call these 'party-pleasers'. Just wait until you see the look on your dinner guests' faces when you serve these up!

Reduce bloating with potatoes

Potatoes are often put in the category of foods that make you fat due to their carbohydrate content. Carbohydrates are found in bread, oats, pasta, rice, fruits, honey, sweets, chocolate, alcohol and all vegetables, but most people don't overeat carbs from vegetables. In fact, it is possible to lose weight while eating potatoes. Losing weight comes down to a numbers game: if you are in calorie deficit, you will lose weight.

TOP TIP

Potatoes can cause bloating in some individuals, so here is a life hack. Cooking potatoes the night before and either eating them cold or reheating them allows them time to produce resistant starch that naturally makes them easier to digest. Although there are supplements you can take that have these beneficial micro-organisms in them, anything you can do to improve your gut health naturally is always a good idea. I'll take potatoes fried in extra virgin olive oil with poached eggs and greens seasoned with salt over a tablet any day.

Sweet or white potatoes?

Both sweet and white potatoes are good and they have nearly identical calories. There are three main differences between sweet and white potatoes. First, white potatoes are from the nightshade family and sweet potatoes are from the morning glory family. For most people this is of no importance, but in rare cases people have allergies to specific nightshade vegetables. Other foods from the nightshade family include peppers, aubergines and tomatoes. If you think you have an issue with adding in any of these nightshade family vegetables, then sweet potatoes would be the better option for you.

Another difference is that a regular potato is a tuber and a sweet potato is a root. Have you ever left potatoes in a bag for too long only to see them sprouting shoots? The potatoes have been in the dark for so long that they think that they're in the ground. Sweet potatoes, on the other hand, are grown from sweet potato cuttings, which are much harder to grow.

The third difference between sweet potatoes and white potatoes is their antioxidants. I've already mentioned in this book that the darker the colour of a veg, the higher its antioxidant content. Sweet potatoes have higher levels of beta carotene (which is converted into vitamin A in the body) and vitamin C, while white potatoes have higher amounts of potassium. If you're looking to increase the amounts of vitamins A and C in your diet though, sweet potatoes shouldn't be the first thing to add. Greens are much lower in calories and help you to feel full without the heavy, bloated feeling you can get from a high-carb meal. For minimal calories, reach for chard, kale, spinach rocket or parsley to boost your vitamin A and C intake. Green power!

Buying, cooking and growing potatoes

Always buy locally grown organic potatoes; it's not much good buying spuds with an 'organic' logo on them that have been shipped halfway round the world. My cooking tip is to cut, slice or dice your potatoes before steaming or oven-cooking them. This more than halves the cooking time and prevents snacking (which often happens if meals take too long to cook). Quick, efficient cooking is key to achieving any fitness goal: no matter how much people might say they like cooking, you can be sure they prefer eating.

One of the reasons potatoes have been grown in Ireland for hundreds of years is that they can be grown from seed – or even just left in the shed until ready to plant. Traditionally, the planting season starts on 17 March – St Patrick's Day.

Salad greens – top of the list

It's difficult to suggest one single best thing to do for your health, but eating salad greens has to be right up there. In fact, the only reason salad greens aren't top of my list of healthy vegetables is that the list looks best in alphabetical order!

The colour of fruits and vegetables (including greens) is linked with nutrition and with antioxidants in particular. Antioxidants prevent excessive stress on the body and not only reduce ageing and wrinkles, but also increase energy levels. If you have more energy, you are much more likely to train; and when you train, you are able to change your body composition. Have you ever heard the phrase 'Eat the rainbow'? Well, when you eat salad greens, you get the whole spectrum of colours. It's just that green is such a strong colour that it overpowers the others.

Benefits of salads

The advantage of adding these greens to any of your meals is that they are packed full of nutrients such as vitamins C, A and K, iron, magnesium and calcium. As with any vegetable, the nutritional value of salad greens starts to decline the second you harvest them, so buy as fresh as possible. And if you want to look and feel healthier, get on the organic greens! A lot of us know that greens are beneficial for us, but getting them into our diet is half the battle. Hopefully some of the buying, cooking and growing tips below will persuade you to do so.

Buying, cooking and growing salads

Once you taste fresh salad greens that actually have flavour and don't turn to mush at the end of the bag after a few days, you will never go back. Go to markets where you can get your hands on greens that were harvested that morning, with the moisture still on the leaves. Make sure, of course, that you buy organic salads – the fresher the better. Salad greens are in season all year round, with different varieties at different times. They come in many forms, from butterhead soft leaves to the dark leafy greens found in rocket mizuna, baby spinach, chard, kale (see earlier in this chapter) and, one of my favourites, claytonia (a really meaty, heart-shaped, salad green).

Eating nutrient-dense, leafy greens will help increase your health wealth. The key is to make them tasty. My tip is to add greens like spinach to curries or to place them on the plate first, so they take on the flavour of the rest of your meal. Adding leafy greens to your stir-fry will add nutrition, fibre and crunch to your diet (the last of these being important in instructing your stomach to produce leptin, the satiety hormone, to let you know that you're full).

The salad greens that I highly recommend growing and eating include any of the brassica family greens, rocket/arugula, mizuna, pak choi and, for higher anti-oxidants, red frills. These are all related to broccoli. All of these greens are cold-tolerant, and with good reason: there are pests that will prick tiny holes in your salad leaves if you grow them at the wrong time of year.

You can grow salad greens pretty much all year round with little or no backbreaking work. Cold-tolerant greens will even flourish in winter, when winter salads are especially important in your diet as a sub-stitute for broccoli, to which they are related.

All you need to grow your own is a shallow flat tray, a small amount of compost and some seeds. In September, start sowing winter greens seeds (red and green frills and tatsoi are my favourites) in trays or small pots, to be transplanted into the ground two weeks later. Harvest in another two to three weeks. Yes, it's that easy. Just make sure to water them, even at weekends. Plants don't take days off. You can also grow leafy salad greens from the brassica family for the warmer months, but then you can also benefit from other brassica vegetables such as radishes, cauli-flower, cabbage, and, of course, broccoli.

Micro-greens

These are small, immature plants that can be sown and harvested in as little as ten days. These greens make the Organic Fitness Foods list because they can have higher antioxidants than the fully mature plant. They can be pretty expensive to buy and are used in high-end restaurants as a garnish, so there's another incentive to grow your own. A packet of seeds doesn't cost a fortune and they can be grown on your windowsill, so you can have your own fresh, high-antioxidant greens at your fingertips to add to your organic eggs or smoothies in the morning.

It's always best to maximise the benefits of nearly everything we do, so growing a purple broccoli micro-green variety does exactly that. Being purple, it has the same antioxidants as blueberries. They improve your brain function and are a heck of a lot cheaper than blueberries, especially when you grow your own.

Squash – the 'forgotten' vegetable

Squash, for some reason, seems to get forgotten. (Since it develops from the flower-producing part of a plant, squash is botanically a fruit, but most people think of it as a vegetable, which is why it's included in this chapter.) Squash is originally from America and was introduced to my family by an aunt who spent time in Long Island, New York. A pumpkin is a type of squash, but the kind that we typically see at Halloween is not the best for eating flavour-wise.

Squash can be found in all shapes and colours from small to large, yellow to green, short to long and narrow to wide. My favourite variety is Crown Prince, because it's the sweetest squash I've ever tasted. Crown Prince squash is light blue with dark orange flesh on the inside.

Benefits of squash

The flesh is where most of this vegetable's benefits are, and the orange colour indicates – you guessed it – the presence of the antioxidant beta carotene. You'll remember that beta carotene helps make vitamin A, which improves our complexion.

Buying, cooking and growing squash

You will only be able to buy Crown Prince in the winter months (as that's when it comes into season), which makes it perfect for Christmas and even the January health buzz.

Put the whole squash in a 180°C oven for an hour and a half (with your Sunday roast?) and you'll have a nutrient-rich, fibre-dense starter or side dish with any meal. Don't even cut it! The leftovers make a great accompaniment to a salad lunch the following day. Just add in a protein source and greens of any description and you're on to a winner: Monday health lunch sorted.

Squash is often included in beginner starter growing packs because it will grow anywhere. Sow seeds in May, 2cm deep and on their side so that water does not sit on the outer coating and cause them to rot, preventing gemination. Transplant out when the plants are big enough to fend for themselves, 1m apart.

Crown Prince or Golden Bear make a great storable crop packed full of vitamin C, which is great for the immune system during the winter months. And, unlike most other veg, squash gets sweeter in storage.

Yacon – the new superfood?

Yacon is a vegetable that most people haven't heard of, but mark my words: it's going to be the new superfood. (The term 'superfood' gets thrown around a lot, but in my interpretation any food that you are currently not eating and contains the vitamins or minerals you are deficient in is a superfood.)

Yacon is a plant related to the sunflower family, which becomes evident when you see its flower. It attracts bees, so it's the plant that keeps on giving. It comes from South America originally, but (perhaps surprisingly) it can easily be grown in Ireland and the UK. It's a bit like a potato, in that the edible part grows under the ground. Yacon differs from potatoes, however, in that it doesn't get blight. (If we'd only known that, it could have saved us from the Potato Famine…)

Yacon, also called 'ground apple', has a sweet taste, similar to a pear. When yacon is just harvested, it's extremely refreshing. It's full of water, like a melon with crunch. When its leaves emerge, a yacon plant resembles a tall shrub or bush. The leaves are used to make a caffeine-free tea. There's nothing wrong with caffeine in moderation, but it does affect our nervous system and negatively affects our sleep. Sleep, of course, is one of the pillars to optimum health (see Chapter 11), making it even more important to get your hands on some yacon tea-leaves at a country market or grow this flawless crop yourself.

Benefits of yacon

Yacon contains several vitamins and has a high water content – especially important in the winter months, when we typically don't drink enough. It also has anti-inflammatory properties and a type of fibre called inulin, which naturally improves your gut health. Possibly best of all, yacon contains a type of sugar called – wait for it – fructo-oligosaccharides. This fancy-sounding sugar allows you to enjoy a sweet taste without any effect on your blood sugar. This makes yacon a perfect snack for diabetics or people who don't want to have cravings later in the day after eating high-sugar fruit such as dates. I am often asked, 'What the best organic food is to eat?' My answer is, 'The one you're currently not eating,' so give yacon a go!

Buying, cooking and growing yacon

Yacon can sometimes be bought at markets, but to guarantee availability, grow your own. Unlike potatoes, yacon can't be grown from a tuber seed. It has to be grown from a growth spur (a knobbly bit on the end of the stem). To get your hands on one, you need to know someone who already grows them.

These growth spurs are available after harvesting the yacon, so get your growth spur before or just after Christmas so that you can plant it outdoors the following spring, after the last frost. Meanwhile, keep it in moist sand or soil in a pot out of the elements, eg, in your shed. When planting, if you can get more than one, keep them 1m apart.

8
Organic Fitness Foods: Fruits, Herbs & Spices

I n this chapter, we look at the benefits of fruits, how to cook, buy and grow them, and then move on to the benefits of organic herbs and spices.

An apple a day...

Apples are the most commonly consumed fruits in the world, as well as one of nature's most nutritious foods – but not all apples are equal.

Benefits of apples

Apples are also one of nature's natural prebiotics, each one containing 4 grams of your daily goal of

25-30 grams. They are also a good source of immune, system-boosting vitamin C as well as containing smaller amounts of vitamins A, E and B, which improve eye, skin and brain function. Apples are also a great source of beneficial microbes (found on the skin of fresh, raw fruit and veg). Bitter (green) apples are better for digestion (increasing stomach acid), but both sweet and red apples will benefit your gut health. In a study carried out in Austria in 2019 comparing conventional and organic apples, there was a significant difference in the amount of microbiota each contained, with organic apples having far more.[33]

Another significant finding of this study was that there were fewer seeds found in the conventional apple, indicating the presence of fewer antioxidants. Antioxidants are linked to flavour, which is one reason why an organic apple is generally sweeter to the taste. It's important to note that, when grown commercially, apples can be sprayed heavily with harsh chemicals during the growing season, which negates the full benefits to our gut health. Apples are one of the fruits I highly recommend consuming in organic form, either from your own garden or from country markets. In fact, one of the easiest and most sustainable and beneficial things you can do to improve your health is to eat local, fresh organic apples.

Nature has a clever way of providing fruit at certain times of the year in order for them to be of maximum benefit. For example, apples contain potassium, which regulates fluid in the body, as well as having a high percentage of water in its flesh. Eating apples is a way of getting more liquids into your diet in the colder months, as people tend not to drink as much water at this time of the year. Apples are over 80% water. The remainder is made up of carbohydrates, fibre and much smaller amounts of protein and fats. The old adage, 'An apple a day keeps the doctor away' is more than fitting for this fruit.

Buying, cooking and growing apples

Commercial apple crops can be sprayed up to ten times in a growing season, which is why apples are high on the list of foods I strongly recommended buying organic (see The Dirty Dozen™ and The Clean 15™ in Chapter 5). The best way to buy apples is when they are in season. Apples come into season in the cooler months. Definitely buy them from the same country they are grown in as well. Like all fruit and veg, buying apples at a market is your best option. Biting into a soft apple from the summer market is like putting on a wet sock – it serves a purpose, but it's not exactly what you want. Apples can be cooked for making one of my favourite deserts (apple crumble with ground almonds, oats and coconut oil for the top and a huge dollop of organic Greek yoghurt instead of cream), as well as added to a breakfast smoothie or even as a snack with your favourite nut butters.

If you plant your own apple trees (either in a pot or in a sunny, south-facing spot in the garden or allotment), you can enjoy fresh hand-picked apples. Buy fruiting trees at the tail-end of the winter months so that you can plant them in January. New Year, new you. There are literally hundreds of varieties of apples that you can grow. One interesting variety is the Rosette apple. It has pink flesh inside instead of the typical white. What is the significance? You guessed it: it's the antioxidants.

Brilliant berries

Berries not only taste great; they also improve your skin complexion and can increase your energy. Yes, berries are medicine. Many of the benefits of berries are down to the added vitamins and minerals that are in single-ingredient, whole foods. Antioxidants play a big role, too. Remember, the darker the colour of a fruit or vegetable, the more antioxidants it contains. With a lot of people eating pale white foods (white pasta, white bread, white potatoes, white rice), it makes sense to add colourful foods to your diet with fruit, and especially vegetables. Whether it's the anthocyanins that make blackberries black, the beta-carotene that makes carrots and peppers orange or the lycopene that makes tomatoes red, incorporate some of these foods into your diet if you want to improve your health.

Benefits of berries

Berries are the healthiest fruits due to their colours, a distinct indicator of their health benefits. These fruits have bright colours to attract animals to help disperse their seeds. These same colours that attract the animals are the antioxidants that make berries superfoods. Berries are second only to herbs and spices for the number of antioxidants they contain. They generally have nearly ten times more antioxidants than any other fruits or vegetables. Organic berries have higher antioxidants than conventional ones, so to get the most benefits from berries, go for organic.

The berries that contain the highest amounts of antioxidants are blueberries and blackberries. These berries have an abundance of compounds called flavonoids. Flavonoids are a class of polyphenols, a type of antioxidant that is also found in other food items I recommend, such as extra virgin olive oil. The most abundant flavonoid found in dark-coloured berries is anthocyanin, which has the ability to improve your memory.[34] (If only I'd known this when I was in college!)

The most significant vitamins found in berries are vitamins C and K. We know that vitamin C is good for us. Half of us were fed vitamin C tablets growing up and are still taking them today, but I'd much rather have fresh berries than a tablet with my breakfast in the morning. Vitamin C is used by the body to repair cells (muscles, skin cells, etc) and also plays a huge role in developing a strong immune system. Vitamin K aids in blood clotting and wound healing and also aids in forming a protein for stronger bones. There are studies that suggest that people who don't consume enough vitamin K have the highest incidence of bone breakages.[35] As someone who broke both hands growing up, I can tell you that I did not eat half as many vitamin K-rich foods as I should have. Dark leafy greens are packed with vitamin K and they now end up in my kale and berry smoothies.

One handful of berries contains over 50% of your daily manganese requirements.[36] Manganese may not be the most commonly known mineral, yet it has an important role in the body: to send signals to the brain. Simply put, berries are brain food. Manganese is useful in reducing the symptoms of premenstrual syndrome (PMS), which include cramps, food cravings and mood swings. Vitamin K can help regulate hormones, too. Manganese is particularly important to diabetics, as it is used in regulating blood sugar levels, with deficiencies leading to reduced insulin production. As it is also used in the formation of cartilage, one of the first signs of manganese deficiency is joint pain. These are all reasons why berries are on the Organic Fitness Food list.

TOP TIP

Berries are said to be Nature's candy in handy, bite-sized colourful balls. They have to be good for us, right? Well, yes, but nature has made berries small for a reason: they contain natural sugars that, if eaten in excess, can make you store surplus body fat by raising blood sugar and insulin levels. Berries typically come into season at the end of summer, which is Nature's way of providing us with extra body fat going into the winter.

Nowadays though, we can have strawberries, blueberries and raspberries on any day we like (but as ever, I recommend buying in season and locally). Although they have less fructose than some tropical fruit, eating excessive amounts of berries can also cause unpleasant symptoms, from bloating and cramps to diarrhoea due to an excess of sugar. Even natural sugars cause the gut to become porous and leak, leading to symptoms of irritable bowel syndrome (IBS).

Buying, cooking and growing berries

It is worth noting that berries are among the top twelve most heavily sprayed foods (see The Dirty Dozen™ in Chapter 5), so it's best to get them organic or grow your own to prevent any negative effects from chemicals.

Since you shouldn't eat too many of them, combine berries with other in-season organic ingredients. I'm a fan of kale and berry smoothies with a chilled yoghurt and maca powder, flax seeds (omega-3 +

fibre) and your preference of organic protein supplement. Alternatively, combine them with greens in a smoothie: you'll get higher fibre, which can slow down the sugar spike in your blood.

I highly recommend growing fruit bushes. Even if you only have one square metre spare in your garden, you can still plant fruit bushes (preferably in the full sun to ripen the fruit quicker and for the plant to thrive). With minimal effort you could have raspberries, redcurrants, blackcurrants, white currants and strawberry plants and have the freshest fruit at your fingertips. Yes, I did just say not to eat too much of them, but when you grow your own you will see the time and difficulty involved in picking an abundance of fruit. This is the way Nature works.

Tomatoes – nature's love apples

Fresh summer tomatoes are my favourite fruit. Tomatoes can come in all shapes and sizes, from beefy (a fist-sized fruit) to plum and cherry, and in different colours too, but the best ones are the red ones. Those of you who don't care for tomatoes should try home-grown ones – they're a game-changer. In fact, when I first set up a small business growing organic fruit and vegetables, I found tomatoes one of the most enjoyable ones to grow. I grew fifteen different varieties one year, including yellow, orange, purple, red and even green. (Yes, some fully ripe tomatoes are green.)

Selling tomatoes in my first year to restaurants and cafes, I was frequently told that 49c was the current price for supermarket tomatoes (non-organic, that is). I let prospective customers taste a store-bought tomato and then one of my organic tomatoes. This typically sealed the deal. The taste makes all the difference and I can tell you I didn't sell them for anywhere close to 49c a punnet!

The benefits of tomatoes

The many benefits from tomatoes include fibre, vitamin C and lycopene, the antioxidant that gives them their distinctive red colour, adding to the benefits of tomatoes being a natural mood improver. Tomatoes can also help to protect your body from the sun, which is at its most dangerous in the summer months when tomatoes come into fruit. (Great timing again, Mother Nature.) Tomatoes are a brilliant fruit for repairing your skin. Tomatoes and their juices can be used for healing sunburn with their high vitamin C content. This is not an excuse to go out and get sunburnt, but to illustrate how food is medicine for specific times of the year.

Buying, cooking and growing tomatoes

When choosing tomatoes, make sure to pick the best shades of red as these indicate the highest amounts of lycopene. A powerful antioxidant, lycopene has twice the benefits of beta-carotene (the orange-coloured antioxidant found in orange tomatoes). It has the ability to reduce stress, speed up recovery, improve skin health and prevent chronic illness.

The vitamin C content of tomatoes is at its highest concentration in the fluid around the seeds, which has also been proven to prevent illnesses like heart disease and strokes,[37] so make sure not to leave half of the good stuff on the chopping board. One way to avoid this is to get your hands on a variety of tomatoes called Iris. This particular tomato is unique in that its contents don't all spill out when you cut it.

Eating fresh tomatoes is something I look forward to every year, but there is always a glut of them mid-summer. What do you do with them? Juiced organic tomatoes make a nice drink after a training session on a hot day. It will aid in muscle recovery, too, with vitamin C helping to repair the cells (muscle tissue) you have damaged that day. Tomatoes can even be frozen and put into stews in the winter months.

Fresh tomatoes are a treat, but they can be even made better and healthier if you cook them. Using olive oil to increase the absorption of lycopene is one way to maximise the benefits of these fruits. If you're looking to make a healthy sauce for any dish, put a large organic tomato, some fresh basil and a sprinkle of pink Himalayan salt in a pan. This will not only add a serious amount of flavour to your meal, but also eliminates that added sugar which is typically found in jars of tomato sauce. Single-ingredient foods are what the body runs best off.

To grow tomatoes, sow a seed in February. (I sow mine on Valentine's Day each year, as I love tomatoes!) Tomato seeds are tiny. Start them off either on a heated bench in a glasshouse or on a warm windowsill – they have to be at least 21°C to germinate, which is warmer than most seeds need to be. The plant can then grow up to 15ft tall if you let it or have the space in your polytunnel. Otherwise, it can be trained to any size you want. It doesn't start to produce edible fruit until July. It's a long wait, but well worth it.

Herbs

As we've seen, fruit and vegetables are good for you in all kinds of ways, but herbs are even healthier for you due to their higher antioxidant content per serving. My top five herbs are:

1. Oregano

2. Parsley

3. Basil

4. Lemon balm

5. Mint

Include these herbs in your meals to make them even heathier. For example, sprinkle oregano on your pizza – which, of course, you'll make with whole-grain dough, organic mozzarella, your own chemical-free tomatoes and some basil. You can also spice your oats with 5-10 grams of herbs and add them to hot water as a warm drink or to any dish.

Lemon balm and mint in particular make excellent warm drink alternatives to coffee and tea and have little or no negative effects on your sleep. In fact, they have the opposite effect. Having a warm mint tea (whether it be peppermint or fresh mint from your kitchen herb garden) also aids digestion, especially after dinner, allowing the body to relax and improving sleep quality. Oregano, lemon balm and mint are all are easily grown in a bed or pot close to your back door.

Parsley

Parsley is a 'super-green' for several reasons. The antioxidants found in parsley are called lutein and zeaxanthin. They increase blood flow to the back of the eye for improved concentration without the caffeine that can have a negative effect on your sleep. Parsley can be added to smoothies. I make a dairy-free rice smoothie with parsley that is ideal for those who don't tolerate lactose. It contains a total of 40 grams protein, 20 grams fat, 60 grams carbohydrates and 563 calories (a video demonstrating how to make it can be found on my YouTube channel). These are the ingredients:

- 40g oats
- 30g (one scoop) rice protein
- 150g parsley
- 15g flax seeds
- 15g chia seeds
- 200g plant-based milk

If you're not into smoothies, just put some parsley leaves in a cup, add hot water and you have parsley tea without the micro-plastics that are found in some teabags.

Parsley is my favourite herb to grow. It can be bought in a pot, but is easily sown from seed. Sow them in March (three to four seeds per cell or yoghurt tub) and transplant six weeks later, 20cm apart. Harvest the outer leaves and more shoots will emerge from the centre. Although you have to re-sow parsley each year, it will continue to give you greens packed full of antioxidants for a full twelve months if you look after it. Re-sow fresh seeds in spring to keep them fresh.

Basil

Basil should definitely be included in your diet, not only because it goes well on a pizza, with pasta or in a pesto, but also for its health benefits. Basil is an adaptogen herb, meaning that it helps the body to deal with stress (physical, chemical or biological). Stress can come from work, breathing in toxic fumes from traffic, training or anxiety. Adaptogen herbs can help reduce the 'fight or flight' response in the body, which is typically due to an increase of the stress hormone cortisol in the bloodstream. Of course, there is medicine that can reduce stress on the body, but I view foods as medicine and am inclined to try a natural approach first, especially since they taste so good.

Basil is one of my Organic Fitness Foods because, believe it or not, it can have nearly ten times the number of antioxidants than vegetables. Basil is in the Top 10 antioxidant herbs with a 67,553 ORAC score (Oxygen Radical Absorbance Capacity).[38] (The other nine, by the way, are – in no particular order – peppermint, nutmeg, oregano, coriander, parsley, thyme, sage, rosemary and lemon balm.)

As you know, antioxidants help plants defend themselves from pests, insects and strains of bacteria in the soil and the air. We gain the benefits of these antioxidants when we consume basil leaves, benefiting from their immune-boosting properties and their power to neutralise free radicals. The two main types of antioxidants found in basil are orientin and viceninare. These particular antioxidants help protect white blood cells and improve immunity. Basically, they prevent us from getting sick. Basil to the rescue, I say! Add the herb dry or fresh to salads, to Mediterranean dishes or even to a spiced bowl of oats for breakfast.

Basil seeds can be potted 1cm deep in a shallow 7cm pot, with four to five seeds per pot. Sow in April or May for an early crop. Basil originally comes from Italy and other Mediterranean countries and needs plenty of heat in a glasshouse, polytunnel or at least a warm windowsill to grow successfully.

How not to kill your potted basil

Have you ever bought a pot of basil from a super-market, picked off all its leaves, left it on the kitchen windowsill and then wondered why it dies? Like any plant, it needs its leaves to make food for itself, so if you pick them all off, you're consigning the poor plant to an early deathbed (pun intended).

To prolong the life of your basil plant, the secret is to harvest only the top two leaves at a time. This encour-ages the plant to produce two more side stems, giving you four more leaves to harvest. If you want to make a pesto sauce, you'll need several plants. Make sure to water them, too.

Spices

You can't grow spices, but I strongly recommend add-ing them to your diet on account of – you've guessed it – their high antioxidant content. Here are my top five organic fitness spices:

1. Cinnamon

2. Cloves

3. Cayenne pepper

4. Ginger

5. Turmeric

Cinnamon

Cinnamon is not just for Christmas desserts, but can (and should) be used daily. Cinnamon is one of the top five antioxidant spices. It can be easily incorporated into a variety of dishes by sprinkling into oats or on sweet potato brownies or making a cinnamon tea, which has both medicinal properties and a delicious, soothing flavour. Pan-fried pears with a high-protein yoghurt and cinnamon is a favourite dessert of mine.

The medicinal properties of cinnamon include controlling your blood sugar levels (which is why I recommend sprinkling a bit of cinnamon into anything you're having that contains sugar, even natural sugars from fruit), reducing your bad cholesterol and reducing inflammation in the body (which is the root cause of many illnesses).[39]

TOP TIP

A final fitness tip: add cinnamon to your fruit, as it controls your blood sugar levels. And cinnamon is super high in antioxidants in itself, so it's a win-win combination!

Cloves

As a teenager I had an unfortunate experience with cloves, unknowingly biting into some that were buried under a huge plateful of Christmas dinner. If you've ever done the same, you will know that they have a distinctive, almost numbing taste. This is due to their antimicrobial and antifungal properties, which are not the only healthy benefits they give you.

Cloves naturally whiten your teeth, resulting in less plaque and cleaner looking teeth. (They were used for mouth cleaning and treating toothaches long before toothbrushes and toothpaste were invented.) Cloves also have anti-inflammatory properties, reducing the swelling of cells in your body. When even minor natural inflammation occurs, anti-inflammatory foods like cloves help speed up recovery. When the body is under a lot of stress (work, relationships, finances, etc) and we feed ourselves inflammatory foods (sugar, cheap vegetable oils, refined carbohydrates, excess alcohol, poor quality meats, etc), excess inflammation can occur. This can lead to more serious illnesses such as cancer. Adding cloves to your diet can make a huge difference in your overall health.

Introduce cloves into your diet gradually, as they are an acquired taste. I suggest starting by making a warm tea drink with hot water, two to three cloves and a sprinkle of cinnamon (two birds, one stone…) first thing in the morning to hydrate yourself. The antioxidants in the cloves will reduce stress, increasing your energy levels so that you can be more productive in your day.

Cayenne pepper

Cayenne pepper is one of my top five spices for a number of reasons. First, it is a way of adding super flavour to a meal instead of using salt. Second, cayenne pepper has the ability to improve circulation. Improved blood flow results in greater energy, as oxygen and every vitamin from the fresh organic foods you are now eating is carried in the blood to your muscles, helping them to function at optimal levels.

Cayenne pepper not only has beneficial healing properties when ingested, but also when applied topically to wounds. It can speed up the healing of open cuts or scratches, quickly stopping the bleeding and aiding the formation of a scab. It has also long been used for treating headaches and migraines, but of course it's best to get to the source of why you're getting headaches in the first place. (For most people, they're due to dehydration – not drinking enough water.) As all vegetables are extremely high in water, if you season them with cayenne pepper you can prevent headaches while avoiding painkillers, which can become addictive, not to mention the negative effects they can have on your liver.

A word of warning: cayenne pepper is a super-spicy chilli that rates high on the Scoville Scale (this measures the 'heat' of chilli peppers), so be sure to pace yourself when incorporating it in your diet. I know someone who, in an effort to maximise the benefits of cayenne pepper, covered her entire meal with it. I received a phone call requesting emergency assistance – with a six-pack of yoghurt!

Ginger

Ginger is another spice that should definitely be included in your diet. Ginger also has strong anti-inflammatory properties due to its high levels of antioxidants. Before I changed my diet, I used to have poor skin health, with eczema rashes on the back of my arms and legs. These have now completely gone – with no small thanks to ginger.

Ginger also helps reduce gas. (This might be useful information, now that you've been inspired to increase your consumption of organic fruit and veg!) Ginger has also been proven to be more effective for indigestion than some of the best over-the-counter medications.[40] The digestive benefits of ginger are due to its fibre content. Ginger root is a prebiotic fibre, which aids in naturally increasing your good gut bacteria. Ginger has also been found to be as effective as ibuprofen in relieving menstrual pain.[41]

Ginger can simply be chopped and added to stir-fries or curries. You can also make a tea with diced ginger root and warm water or add it to smoothies. (Recipes for Sweet Chia Green Smoothie and Organic Apple & Cinnamon Smoothie can be found on my YouTube channel.)

Turmeric

Turmeric is *the* super-spice when it comes to improving your overall health. Turmeric benefits your heart function and fitness and is great for reducing muscle aches and pains. The beneficial antioxidant in turmeric is curcumin, which gives it its distinctive orange colour. One study found that consuming turmeric – and curcumin antioxidants in general – was as beneficial to your health as an hour of training.[42] Turmeric must, however, be consumed with black pepper in order to activate the curcumin. So, whether you want relief from Delayed Onset Muscle Soreness (DOMS) after you work out, or just relief from a common knee or lower back pain, adding turmeric to your diet can be of benefit.

One of my favourite benefits of turmeric is that it can boost your brain-derived neurotrophic factor (BDNF). BDNF is a protein that helps the brain to function at optimal levels. BDNF can help in retaining newly-received information, as well as improving memory. When you start to eat more of the foods that can improve your body physically and mentally, you become a healthier version of you. Foods that benefit the brain are important, and BDNF-boosting turmeric has been proven to decrease depression. The fibre from the turmeric root will also improve the health of your gut, where 90% of our serotonin is produced.[43]

Add turmeric to curries, stir-fries and even my Organic Fitness Smoothies. A word of caution when cutting fresh turmeric – it can stain your hands to make you look like a smoker.

Summary

Hopefully, I have given you enough information and encouragement to go out and buy more fruit and veg and incorporate them into your diet. You will know by now that organic fruit and vegetables contain higher amounts of antioxidants than conventionally grown ones. This basic nutritional tip should give you the knowledge to reach for darker-coloured foods the next time you're shopping. With any of the foods that are mentioned in this book, however, adding one food item or eating organic for a few days isn't going to dramatically change your life; the incremental effect it will have over time will. Trust me.

9
Organic Fitness Foods: Other Foods

In this chapter, I'll look at some other organic fitness foods (including meat and dairy products), as well as at supplements (I don't mean the kind you pop in pill form, but natural food supplements).

Meat, fish and dairy products

We looked at meat, fish and dairy products in Chapter 1 when we discussed protein sources. It's worth repeating here that all these foods are best eaten organic. Eating organic animal protein will prevent excess antibiotics and growth hormones being consumed, as their use is prohibited by registered organic meat producers. Organically raised animals must also be grass-fed, which means that all the natural vitamins from the soil are transferred to the meat.

There are both pros and cons to consuming meat. Meat is nutrient-dense, with easily absorbed iron and vitamin B12, which has an effect on your energy levels. On the other hand, poor-quality meat typically served in fast food restaurants and other 'convenience' foods comes from animals that have often been fed growth hormones, grazed on sprayed land or never even laid a hoof on grass. Non-organic meats can also contain antibiotics. Another important point is that it can take nearly 100 times as much water to produce 1 kilogram of animal protein as it does to produce the same amount of vegetable protein,[44] but remember that you can't achieve optimal health on a diet of vegetables alone without supplements (see later in the chapter).

Fish can be a good source of healthy fats (mackerel, sardines and salmon are all high in omega-3) and are a good source of selenium, which is good for an under-active thyroid – although a single Brazil nut contains more than your daily recommended amount of selenium. The problem is that with the oceans becoming increasingly polluted with micro-plastics, these fish are increasingly given feed to brighten their skin. In a natural setting, this would indicate higher nutrition in the fish, but not in this case. Take salmon: the reddish-pink colour of their skin comes from antioxidants in their feed, whereas in the wild, salmon eat algae and other small crustacea.

White fish (less fatty) such as haddock, hake, cod, bass and tilapia are also high in protein and are often a better option if you are looking to reduce the calories in your meals, especially as they are usually more sustainably farmed. When buying in a supermarket, look out for a blue logo marked Marine Stewardship Council (MSC), a non-profit organisation that works to end overfishing around the world.

Yoghurts and cheese are both natural probiotics that improve your gut health and can be beneficial to people who can tolerate the lactose in milk products, but again, not all food is created equally and when non-organic animals are given unnecessary antibiotics these can have negative effects on our gut. Choosing the right protein foods is key for optimal health.

Excellent eggs

There is a lot to be said for starting your day with eggs. They are a complete protein, they contain healthy fats, they are quick to cook and versatile. The egg has an amino acid profile like no other food, containing all nine of the essential amino acids (see Chapter 1) and almost every vitamin, including B12. This is extremely important for the body, especially if you don't consume a lot of meat. B12 is involved in the development of red blood cells, maintaining a healthy nervous system and normal brain function. If your diet is void of meat and eggs, you must supplement with vitamin B12.

Another benefit of eggs is that they contain healthy fats, which increase the absorption of the vitamins A, D, E and K found in greens, so adding eggs to a bed of lightly steamed kale gives you the best of both worlds. Eggs, of course, come in two parts: the white and the yolk. Let's look at each in turn:

- **Egg white:** Typically favoured over the yolk, egg white is a high-quality, single-ingredient natural protein source with fewer calories than a whole egg. (Well, you're only eating half of it!) In fact, egg whites are protein and little else, so if you are looking for natural source of protein with a meal, adding egg whites to a stir-fry will bump up your daily intake for the day without increasing the fat content.

- **Egg yolk:** The theory that the cholesterol in egg yolks is a reason not to eat too many of them has been disproved.[45] The cholesterol in egg yolk has no direct link with the cholesterol in your body, most of which is made by the liver. In fact, the yolk is the 'better' half of the egg in that it contains more than half of its nutrients, including the above-mentioned vitamins and amino acids. It also contains selenium (good for thyroid health, especially if you don't eat a lot of fish, meat or other dairy products) and phosphorus (great for repairing muscle cells, especially after exercise).

The yolk also contains half the egg's protein and the healthy fats that people are often told to stay away from.

Antioxidants in eggs

Egg yolks contain the antioxidants lutein and zeaxanthin (derived from the Latin and Greek words for 'yellow'). You'll remember that the darker the colour, the higher the antioxidant content, so eggs with dark orange yolks contain more of these antioxidants. Since lutein and zeaxanthin come from plants, chickens that are grass-fed (ie, free-range) will lay eggs that are higher in antioxidants.

Lutein and zeaxanthin have the ability to improve blood flow to the back of the eye, which helps you concentrate – another way to wean yourself off the sleep-destroyer, coffee – but don't wait until your eyesight gives you trouble to start eating eggs! (Lutein and zeaxanthin are also found in dark, leafy greens such as kale and spinach.)

The three grades of eggs

There are huge and confusing differences between eggs, which may be labelled caged, free-range, free to roam, pasture-raised, organic, natural, enhanced with omega-3, antibiotic-free… The list goes on. Let's look at the three main grades more closely:

- **Cage eggs:** These are typically the cheapest and come from hens that are kept in cages. Not only is this unethical, but the best nutrition can't come from animals that can't exercise and often never see daylight, which gives eggs their vitamin D. Cage eggs also typically have less healthy fats (omega-3 and omega-6). You (don't) get what you (don't) pay for.

- **Free-range eggs:** These eggs come from hens that are allowed to spend at least half of their time outdoors on land that is not registered as organic. Compared with cage eggs, free-range eggs are higher in omega-3 (which is typically the healthy fat we lack), since free-roaming animals get essential healthy fats from eating greens and bugs. These hens can, however, be given antibiotics, so it's worth checking where your eggs come from.

- **Organic eggs:** These differ from free-range in that the hens must be raised on registered organic land (where omega-3 comes from) that is free from the use of harsh chemicals such as glyphosate. Organic hens must not be given routine antibiotics or fed GMO grain. They are fed organic, registered feed, which increases the beneficial antioxidants in the eggs and gives the yolks their distinctive colour and taste.

You don't have to be a registered organic farmer to produce quality natural, free-ranging/roaming, antibiotic-free omega-3-filled eggs. Keeping your own hens, if you have space for them, can provide you with fresh heathy eggs from well-treated animals, while also giving you great fertiliser for gardening.

Supplements

As children, with parents that always wanted the best for us, my siblings and I took multivitamin tablets containing vitamins C, A and D, magnesium and even omega-3 fish tablets to improve our skin and brain health. I still grew up suffering from poor skin health (rashes, irritation and eczema), mild asthma and severe allergy problems. In addition to taking supplements, I applied creams to try to keep these issues at bay (which was expensive), but every year my nose would run and I would blow it so hard that by the start of summer I looked like Rudolph. Bathing in cool water was the only major relief for the rashes on the back of my legs and arms. If only I knew then what I know now.

Vitamin C is a natural antihistamine and is found naturally in fruits and vegetables, along with other benefits. Adding natural vitamin C to my diet has significantly improved my life. My hay fever and irritable rashes are completely gone, eliminating the need to constantly carry tablets (which were only barely keeping the symptoms at bay) and I no longer use an inhaler before sports or activities (which was previously a must). The only supplements I now take are derived from whole foods and the money I save on supplements and creams, I spend on organic food. Food is medicine.

The definition of a supplement is something that provides what you can't get from your diet. That doesn't have to mean pills. With half of the population taking a daily supplement, people are more often than not missing out when they consume them.[46] Supplements have been said to be able to cure everything from hair loss to cancer, to boost energy and offset the effects of menopause. We are currently bombarded with advertisements on social media for supplements or processed food items labelled 'fortified with vitamins' that will 'improve the health of the nation', but few people extol the nutritional benefits of food that naturally contains iron, magnesium, vitamin C and other nutrients that most people take in tablet or powdered form. (There's little money to be made from people who are healthy…) Here are some foods that can naturally supplement your diet:

Maca

Maca is a superfood for that I take every morning. It is a root vegetable similar in appearance to a stubby parsnip, but actually from the same family as broccoli, kale and cabbage – the brassica family. The maca root is vegan, vegetarian and plant-based friendly. It is native to Peru and comes in a range of colours: red, yellow and black (the most common being yellow).

Benefits of maca

Maca contains high levels of antioxidants, which I've already mentioned one or twice, but remember that each and every vegetable has different antioxidants, with varying health benefits. Maca contains polyphenols and polysaccharides, which have been found to play a part in improving metabolism. This is a key benefit if you are looking to shed a few pounds, but important in any case, as your metabolism is the process by which the body converts the food we eat into energy.

Maca is an excellent source of vitamins: vitamin A (good for sight), vitamin B2 (aids in breaking down protein) and vitamin C (a natural antihistamine). It also contains fibre (a natural mood improver) and some protein too – all things people take supplement tablets for. Maca is also an 'apoptogenic', which is a fancy name for plants and herbs that help the body deal with stress (perhaps from our job, busy schedule or a sickness or illness).

Maca can be used as an energy drink (by adding 5 grams of powder to cold water), but differs from conventional 'energy' drinks. It has no caffeine, no added sugars and no side-effects, such as the jitters that some people get with coffee and commercial energy drinks. People I train report being energised quite soon after starting to take it. Since maca also contains iron, it increases the body's ability to transport oxygen around the body to working muscles, allowing them to function better for day-to-day tasks and improving your performance in training and sports. Increased blood supply also benefits the brain, and I have personally found increased clarity in my thoughts after taking maca.

Post-menopause women with sexual dysfunction and low libido have been found to have an increased sex drive just days after taking maca each morning, when compared with a placebo group.[47] This is because maca balances sex hormones like oestrogen, reducing symptoms such as weight gain and bloating. Another common problem that maca powder can relieve is premenstrual syndrome (PMS), easing tender breasts, upset stomach, headaches, and probably most importantly, mood swings.[48]

In fact, this super vegetable has the capacity to reduce sexual dysfunction and increase sex drive in both men and women. Maca has been shown to increase not only sperm count, but also sexual desire, with increased testosterone levels.[49] (Before you ask, yes, I take it daily: 15 grams in my overnight oats.) Finally, there is evidence that consuming maca can help reduce bad cholesterol levels, which are the leading cause of heart attacks.[50]

Buying and using maca

In Europe, maca typically comes in powdered form, and you can buy it from health food shops or online. It is important to get organic maca to maximise its benefits and flavour: a slightly nutty, butterscotch taste. Take 15-20 grams daily.

You can add it to smoothies or breakfast foods and even make homemade sauces for main meals. I add it to yoghurts, increasing the benefits of the snack tenfold. It has been suggested that maca should be mixed with water or a simple fruit juice and taken on an empty stomach fifteen minutes before breakfast to increase the speed of absorption, but this isn't essential. You will gain the benefits whatever way you add it to your diet.

Cacao

Cacao is the second thing that I take daily and also has numerous benefits. Often confused with cocoa powder as the names are similar, cacao contains no added sugar and is non-dairy. Cacao typically comes in powder or, preferably, block form. It is made from naturally fermented beans using heat from the sun, which is in line with my basic ethos: the less processed the food, the better.

Benefits of cacao

A lot of people eat chocolate to improve their mood and there is science behind this. Chocolate contains cacao, which is a natural prebiotic that produces serotonin (a 'happy hormone'). The benefit of eating chocolate is related to the amount of cacao it contains (along with other ingredients), so read the label and go for a high percentage of cacao and a low percentage of sugar. Aim for 80% or higher and make sure it's organic.

When people say they crave chocolate, what their body is actually craving is magnesium, which is also found in cacao. Cravings are the body's way of signalling that there is a nutrient imbalance, and as we know, magnesium is needed for 300 different processes.

The cacao bean has even higher antioxidants than blueberries, goji berries or red wine. With cacao, as with other foods, the darker the colour, the more antioxidants and the greater the benefits. As you now know, antioxidants improve blood flow, so cacao can naturally boost your brain function, increasing BDNF (a protein discussed earlier). Another benefit of cacao is that it improves blood flow – and you will know the many benefits of that by now. The improvement in circulation is due to the nitric oxide in cacao, which dilates your blood vessels. Nitric oxide is also found in beetroot, chard and rocket greens – all foods I recommend growing or adding to your diet.

Chocolate vs cacao powder

Most chocolate contains sugar (if it didn't, it would be extremely bitter), so by eating raw cacao powder you get its benefits without the negatives from the added sugar. Cacao powder can also be substituted for coffee or other caffeinated drinks because it gives you a similar boost without massively affecting your adrenals. Your adrenals produce the stress hormone cortisol, which gives us alertness, so if you are already stressed and continue to drink copious amounts of high-caffeine drinks, you are not helping the situation. For a natural energy boost at any time of day, make a warm drink with 15 grams cacao, 5 grams cinnamon and 15 g maca powder with a pinch of pink Himalayan salt for natural electrolytes. If you are trying to wean yourself off coffee, give it a try.

Chia seeds and flax seeds

These seeds may be small, but they have big benefits. Chia and flax seeds' main selling point is that they are a great plant-based source of the essential fatty acid, omega-3. If your diet is strictly plant-based and you are looking to increase your intake of omega-3 fats, these seeds are a must. Both chia and flax are also packed with fibre and protein.

Which is better? Chia has higher insoluble fibre, getting things flowing in the morning, so to speak, and removing toxins in the body that we all have no matter how 'clean' our diet is. Chia seeds can be eaten whole or ground, but I recommend steeping them (another addition to your steeped overnight oats). Flax seeds, on the other hand, have a higher omega-3 content than chia and are especially high in a type of fibre called lignans, which helps protect against heart disease and dreaded cancer. So, the answer is both! Add them to smoothies or breakfasts or sprinkle ground flax on salad lunches to get twice the goodness.

Summary

The body wants to heal itself. Every time you eat, you are either helping it or hindering it. Changing to a diet rich in whole organic foods is the best way to help your body do what it is supposed to do and perform at its best. Of course, food isn't the only 'fuel' for your body, so in the next part of this book I'll look at the benefits of exercise as well as sleep, sun, sea swims and saunas.

PART THREE
ORGANIC FITNESS

In the first two parts of this book, I focused on how eating (and drinking) affects your fitness. In Part Three, I turn to other ways of improving your overall fitness. The word 'fitness' tends to conjure up images of gyms and fearsome black machines, sweaty classes and pavement-pounding. It's a lot more than that, involving not only exercise (of course), but also sleep – yes, good sleep is essential to fitness – and sunshine. You can even get fit watching Netflix. If you don't believe me, read on…

10
Exercise

One of the core habits practised by successful people, from me or you all the way up to Mark Zuckerberg, is exercise. In his book *The Power of Habit: Why We Do What We Do in Life and Business*,[51] Charles Duhigg explains how exercising prompts changes in other areas of your life, because how you do anything is how you do everything. If you want to improve at anything, you must be consistent. Training develops self-discipline when performed regularly – whether you go to the gym, work out at home, swim in the sea, run, jog or all of the above. Remember that exercise can also take the form of walking, cycling, swimming and gardening, depending on your fitness goal.

Do you ever wonder what actually happens to your body when you start exercising? What are the physical changes? What happens to your muscles, your heart (a muscle itself) and your mind? These are the types of questions I'm going to answer in this chapter.

Five benefits of exercise

There are lots of benefits of exercise but I've broken them down into five main categories:

1. Physical changes

2. Natural mood improver

3. Improved skin health

4. Improved sleep

5. More brain power

Physical changes

Physical changes such as weight loss, muscle development and a more toned physique are achieved using compound movements that use large muscle groups that tear muscle fibres, and in turn, burn calories. The largest muscle groups of the body are the legs, back, chest and shoulders. Using these muscles is key to maximising your workout time.

Natural mood improver

People who exercise are generally happier. Most of us have heard of serotonin, also known as the 'happy hormone'. Exercise increases the production of serotonin. How does that happen? Tryptophan is an amino acid produced naturally in the body, and a small amount goes to the brain to trigger the production of serotonin. When you exercise, you tear muscle fibres. The body repairs these fibres by sending amino acids to the muscles that need repairing. When this happens, there are fewer amino acids in the bloodstream overall, creating less competition. With less competition, a greater amount of tryptophan reaches the brain, producing higher levels of serotonin.

Tryptophan can be found in larger concentrations in protein foods, including all meats (especially turkey), eggs, peanuts, pumpkin seeds and tofu. Plant-based sources of tryptophan include dark leafy greens, sunflower seeds, soya, pumpkin seeds, mushrooms, broccoli and peas.

Improved skin health

When we exercise at high intensity, we sweat. Some people say that sweat is 'fat crying', but here is some science. We have a daily build-up of toxins in our body from the air we inhale while working out, from breathing the air outside and from the food and drink we consume (especially non-organic). Being the intelligent machine it is, the body can excrete toxins, but only when we sweat. Sweating is induced by daily activities, but is increased when you exercise.

A high percentage of sweat glands are found on your face (a common place for toxins to build up), causing spots or blemishes if you don't sweat. Extremely expensive face creams may claim to improve your complexion, but they can also prevent your skin from breathing and lead to poor skin health. Instead, have a medium to hot shower after your workout and then moisturise your skin after some of the toxins in your body have been removed. I have a general rule that anything applied to my skin (especially my face) must be organic or natural.

Improved sleep

Improved sleep is probably one of the most underrated spinoff benefits of exercise, because without adequate sleep our bodies cannot repair and recover (see Chapter 11). We all know how we feel after a poor night's sleep. Exercise can increase sleep quality by reducing the amount of time it takes to fall asleep – ie, decreasing the amount of time you lie awake in bed. Physical activity can also alleviate daytime sleepiness and, for some people, reduce the need for sleep medication.

Because exercise increases your body temperature and sleep requires your body temperature to reduce by around 1%, exercise just before hopping into bed is not recommended. Exercising well before bedtime gives your body time to brings its temperature back to normal. Conversely, exercising outdoors in the morning exposes you to natural sunlight, which reduces melatonin (the sleep hormone – see Chapter 11 on sleep), so morning exercise increases your wakefulness. That said, there are benefits to exercising at any time of day. Choosing a time that suits you is better than not exercising at all.

More brain power

We all want to be smarter, right? Exercising can help us do just that. Exercise increases the amount of a protein called brain-derived neurotrophic factor (BDNF) produced naturally in the brain. This protein helps you concentrate, as it produces new brain cells in a part of the brain called the hippocampus – part of the brain linked with memory. When the number of cells increases, it improves your brain's ability to retain information. An important point to note is that as we age, BDNF decreases, making it even more important to continue to exercise in whatever way we can as we get older.

Boost your BDNF naturally

Although exercise is the most effective way to boost this protein in the brain, there are other ways to boost BNDF:

- **Food:** Vitamin B3 has been linked with increased BDNF, improves skin health, reduces anxiety, improves your immune system and increases energy (important for exercise).[52] What foods have it? All types of meat contain vitamin B3, but I'm encouraging you to eat more plant-based food and those that are high in B3 include nuts and seeds – specifically, almonds, walnuts and pumpkin seeds. Peanuts (which are a legume), green peas and brown rice are also high in B3.

- **Drink:** I recommend drinking green tea to boost your B3 intake. It has less caffeine than coffee or the latest, brightly-coloured energy drink. It's not that caffeine is bad; it's just that too much of it can negatively affect your sleep, and in turn reduce the production of BDNF.[53] Sleep is one of the pillars of health that improve so many systems in the body (see Chapter 11). Green tea can also improve your immune system (vitamin C) and it contains the antioxidant ECGS, which reduces anxiety. You don't have to buy fancy, expensive teabags that are wrapped in micro-plastics; just have a small pot of mint at your back door that you can pick and add hot water to for a fresh organic drink.

- **Hot and cold exposure:** Saunas, steam rooms, cold showers and sea dips can all boost BDNF, as we'll see later. Whether it's exposure to heat or cold, the extreme temperature change increases your heart rate, which in turn increases blood flow to the brain. Increased volumes of blood carry protein to the hippocampus (the part of the brain that increases memory and retains information) in greater quantities.

- **Direct sunlight exposure:** Too many of us jump out of bed, travel to work and sit indoors for eight to ten hours every day. Exposure to direct sunlight early in the morning will lead to an increase in cortisol, which will allow the body to awaken naturally. Cortisol is the stress hormone which we want a small amount of in the morning. An increase in cortisol in the morning also aids sleep that night, which in turn leads to increased BDNF.

Magnesium and exercise

Exercise increases the body's demand for magnesium, which is a mineral that we typically lack in our diet. The recommended intake is between 300 milligrams and 500 milligrams of magnesium per day.[54] Magnesium is used for over 300 functions in the body, one of which is energy production. Good sources of magnesium are dark leafy greens such as kale, spinach, rocket, rainbow chard, cabbage and broccoli. For example, 100 grams of spinach contains around 80 milligrams of magnesium, which is nearly 20% of your daily recommended intake. If you want your body to recover faster, increase your energy and sleep better, eat your greens (a kale omelette or a green maca smoothie come to mind).

The secret of saunas

The benefits of a sauna have been known for centuries, but my own initiation into its secrets came in my late twenties when I went on a skiing trip with a friend. One evening, after hitting the slopes all day, we decided to go for a swim. It was -4°C and deep snow covered the ground. After a bit of gallivanting (sliding down slides, diving into the pool headfirst, etc), we discovered a sauna and headed straight for it. I still remember my blissful state when I re-emerged from it several minutes later. Here are five reasons you should take regular saunas (if you can):

1. **Sweat out toxins:** Taking a sauna makes you sweat, which, as we have seen, has benefits for your body. When you increase your body temperature, you excrete toxins such as bisphenol A (BPA) through your sweat glands. BPA is a toxin that is used to make plastics. It can build up in the body as it cannot be broken down by the metabolism. With food items increasingly being wrapped or stored in plastic containers (even organic products), our exposure to BPA is higher than ever, making it even more important to either grow your own or shop at farmers' markets

or real health food shops that sell in-season fruit and veg. Excessive exposure to BPA can cause childhood asthma (something I suffered with, but now have little or no issue with) and have negative effects on the brain. It has even been linked with illnesses such as Alzheimer's.[55]

2. **Boost BDNF:** As mentioned earlier, BDNF is a protein that helps boost the brain's ability to retain information. It is increased by greater blood flow and saunas increase blood flow.

3. **Speedy recovery:** There is science behind why people use the sauna after a workout. With the increased temperature, your heartrate pumps faster, increasing blood flow, which transports amino acids in the blood to repair your muscles more quickly. This means you'll have fewer aches and pains after a workout and can get back to training those muscles sooner.

4. **Improves endurance:** Research suggests that this increase in blood flow puts the body under stress, mimicking the stress you get during an intense workout session.[56] (To maximise the benefits, I recommend exercising and then having a sauna.)

5. **Increases happy hormones:** Increased blood flow also boosts the amount of tryptophan getting to the brain, which causes dopamine (the 'happy hormone') to be released.

Ice baths and cold-water swims

From one extreme to the other: hot to cold. I put ice baths and cold-water swims in this chapter because they are a form of exercise – even though they are not for the faint-hearted, especially in the winter! The idea of using this form of exercise as a recovery strategy has been around for centuries and has recently increased in popularity, thanks in part to Wim Hof, the Dutch 'Iceman' who holds world records for sitting in ice baths for nearly two hours (which I don't recommend, especially if it's your first time!).[57]

I prefer cold-water dips to ice baths, because I don't live far from the coast and no one minds if you run, jump and splash about in the sea (especially first thing in the morning when no one is around), whereas your neighbours might object to your screaming in your bathtub at 6am! Here are some of the benefits of cold-water swims and ice baths:

1. **Speeds recovery:** When you enter cold water, your heart rate rises, increasing the amount of blood flow in the body, which also increases the flow of proteins and vitamins and minerals around the body, aiding muscle repair. Being in either an ice bath or cold water will also reduce swelling in any area in the body – which is one of the reasons we apply ice packs to an injury; dipping the entire body in ice-cold water maximises the effect.

2. **Helps mental clarity:** When you're exposed to cold water, blood rushes to your brain. Nutrients and oxygen are carried in the blood, which improves your brain function. This gives you a sense of improved attention and focus. That's the science behind why our brain functions better after cold water exposure, but there's another, less 'scientific' reason: when you jump into cold water, it's a shock to the system and wakes you up.

3. **Cold water is colder than our natural body temperature:** This causes the body to work slightly harder to maintain its core temperature. When done regularly, cold-water swimming can make your circulatory system (heart and blood vessels) more efficient.

4. **Benefits skin health:** Sea dips or cold-water exposure from ice baths can increase blood flow to the skin as well. Again, this carries oxygen and nutrients to the skin, removing toxins that build up in our skin from the air we breathe and the pollution we come into contact with.

5. **Improves mood:** The sense of improved mood comes from the essential amino acid, tryptophan, reaching parts of the brain that increase the production of serotonin and dopamine. And when you get out of the water with chattering teeth and warm up with a glass of ginger tea as you dry off, well, how could you not feel happier?

6. **Helps you sleep:** There a several reasons
    seawater promotes sleep and one of them is the
    fact that it contains magnesium. Magnesium
    comes from sea plants such as seaweed, which
    have their own benefits, too, and so should be
    included in your diet. After salt, magnesium is
    the second most prevalent mineral in the sea and
    can be absorbed through the skin.

Stretching and grounding

Stretching is light exercise, and like walking, is too
often overlooked. It can reduce stress and anxiety,
increase flexibility, prevent lower back pain and help
with sleep. Like any other exercise, stretching also
increases blood flow and heart rate (and you know
the many benefits of that by now).

Stretching can reduce stress if you take deep breaths
and hold a stretch for a couple of seconds so that
your heart rate slows. Increased flexibility is a benefit that is often overlooked, especially by people who
are training. Holding a stretch for up to ten seconds
allows the muscles to slowly expand so that you
improve your flexibility. Increased flexibility also
increases your range of motion, which in turn allows
you to tear more muscle fibre and build a stronger,
leaner, more toned physique. When stretching is
incorporated into your daily and weekly routine,
tight back muscles are loosened, which makes it

easier to stand up tall and avoid lower back pain (which is all too common).

When I discovered all this and saw its benefits first-hand, I fitted stretching into my daily routine. Whether you sit at a desk or work outside, incorporating stretching into your day is key to improving your overall health. It doesn't have to be for twenty, thirty or sixty minutes – five minutes of stretching is better than none at all – but the more you do, the greater the benefits.

TOP TIP

Being the kind of guy who likes to maximise the benefits of anything I do, I often combine stretching and grounding. Grounding, as the word suggests, means placing any part of your body – typically your feet and hands – on the ground. This has been proven to increase blood flow and reduce stress levels by neutralising free radicals, so when you combine it with stretching you kill two birds with one stone.[58]

Weights and resistance training

When you train with weights (a kettlebell, dumbbells or bags of sugar) or work with resistance on a muscle (using tension-style trainers or HIIT finishers), you will tear muscle fibres, which helps you burn calories not only during a workout, but also while sitting on the couch. Your body needs to repair these tears using the protein foods you have consumed. This is where you use food to your advantage. Instead of calories from food being used just to fuel the body, you give them another job to do: repairing your muscles.

Adding more resistance by training with weights burns off glycogen stores, which come from carbs – your body's first source of energy. In this way you are tapping into your body's reserves, your body fat, and using it as a direct fuel source. Adding a 'finisher' (an intense burst of cardio at the end of a workout) makes weight loss that bit easier. You can use running too, but I prefer a high-intensity finisher to save time. A finisher I use involves two moves: high knees and jumping jacks (my Organic Fitness Training Program shares more details).

NEAT: Exercise that isn't really exercise

Finally, in this chapter on exercise, a word about the benefits of 'not exercising' – or rather a form of exercise called Non-Exercise Activity Thermogenesis (NEAT), which means burning calories when going about your daily business. This can include walking from place to place, climbing stairs, cooking, cleaning, shopping, toe-tapping and playing an instrument. (Some of these I do better than others!) These activities might not seem like exercise, but let's say you work out for between thirty and sixty minutes a day and sleep for eight hours. That leaves at least fifteen hours of the day for you to burn up calories with NEAT.

You can burn up to 500 calories simply by doing your daily 10,000 steps. You don't have to go to the gym or a class and it's free. NEAT is not a replacement for regular exercise, of course (don't kid yourself), but it's something to focus on. There are several ways in which you can increase your NEAT, which is especially important if you spend most of your day sitting at a desk:

1. We've already looked at the benefits of daily stretching and this can also increase your NEAT.

2. Park your car in the furthest carpark space available at work, when shopping and when going to the gym. Better still, cycle or walk instead of using the car.

3. Take the stairs at any opportunity you get: at work, in carparks, at the theatre, when visiting people in an apartment block and even on holiday.

4. Do regular chores such as cleaning your room and washing your car once a week.

5. Include a walk in your daily routine before or during work or after dinner. Walking increases steps and aids in digestion. I love it when one thing benefits another to maximise advantages in reaching your fitness goals.

Summary

After reading this section of the book, I hope you are motivated to incorporate some form of exercise, including stretching, into your daily routine. There is no doubt that you will feel the benefits, which include greater energy, better concentration and memory, improved sleep, better overall health and greater happiness. Put the word '*Exercise*' in your diary right now!

11
Sleep And Sun

Good sleep and adequate sunlight are two crucial elements in any health and fitness programme. In this chapter, I'll explain why. If you have ever woken up groggy or feeling that you need a kick to get you out of bed, or if you're prone to seasonal affective disorder (SAD), this chapter will help you.

Sleep

Sleep is something we do every single day, yet we often neglect it. Sleep is vital, because this is when our bodies recover. While you're sleeping, your body is busy repairing cells and producing hormones, as well as processing all the information you have been exposed to during the day.

As someone who used to be a poor sleeper, I know from experience that not getting quality sleep can affect everything from energy levels to appetite, concentration, skin, mental health and hormone levels. Sleep allows your muscle tissue to be repaired, helps you maintain a healthy weight, reduces your stress levels and – you'd better believe it – makes you look younger. During sleep, your skin's blood flow increases, rebuilding collagen and repairing damage from excessive UV exposure, thereby reducing wrinkles and age spots. The phrase 'beauty sleep' is, in fact, based in science!

Good sleep also makes you less hungry. Sound odd? Sleep increases the body's production of leptin, the satiety hormone that signals to the brain that you are full. A recent study found that when people got more sleep, they were less hungry and experienced a reduced desire for sweet and salty foods, while a single night of sleep deprivation increased their levels of hunger and ghrelin, the appetite hormone.[59]

You have probably heard that we should sleep for between seven and nine hours. The longest recorded time anyone has spent without sleep is 264 hours – not something I'm advocating. The most sleep-deprived I have ever been was in my late twenties when I went to a seven-day music festival in Budapest, during which I got less than three hours of 'lying down' (I could barely call it sleep) per night. The combination of alcohol and sleep deprivation meant that I came back from the holiday feeling like I needed another holiday.

To appreciate the benefits of sleep, it's important to understand how sleep 'works'.

Sleep broken down

There are two main phases of sleep:

1. Non-REM (non-rapid eye movement)

2. REM (rapid eye movement)

Both describe exactly what happens during that phase: during phase one, your eyes don't move behind your eyelids; during phase two, they move rapidly. Phase two is when we 'imprint' memories of information we took in that day, while during non-REM (which is the phase of deeper sleep) the body unwinds and recovers from exercise done during the day.

When you sleep, you sleep in cycles of approximately ninety minutes. There are three non-REM phases and one REM phase within each ninety-minute cycle. The length of time you spend in non-REM sleep changes through the night. During the first half of the night, you have more non-REM and very little REM. In the second half of the night, you get more REM. An eight-hour sleep generally falls into the following stages:

Stage 1 (Falling asleep): The first stage, the lightest period of sleep, lasts five to ten minutes. Stage 1 is also the easiest to wake up from, which is why power naps are recommended to be twenty minutes or less; this prevents you falling into a deeper sleep and waking up in the middle of it feeling groggy. If you want a longer nap, sleep for an entire ninety minutes to complete a full sleep cycle.

Stage 2 (Light sleep): During this stage, your heart rate slows, your body temperature lowers and an especially important process happens: the information that you have obtained during the day is transferred from the short-term to the long-term memory, where it is consolidated. This is a reason not to stay up all night just before an exam!

Stage 3 (Deeper sleep): This is one of the most restorative periods of sleep, as this is when the body promotes skin and muscle repair. Your breathing rate slows right down and your muscles relax. Another important function that occurs during this cycle is that the body releases the hormone leptin, which aids in appetite control.

Stage 4 (REM sleep): This stage consists mostly of REM sleep, during which vivid dreams occur. The duration of REM sleep varies and can be as long as sixty minutes of the final ninety-minute cycle of your sleep. Blood flow increases to the genitals, which is why REM sleep is also linked with wet dreams.

It is important to understand that good sleep is as much a matter of quality as quantity. You should always try to wake at the end or start of a ninety-minute cycle. If you wake up feeling groggy and unrested, this is often due to waking in the middle of a sleep cycle. When I want to get up at 6am, I go to sleep at 10pm. You can't take any shortcuts with your sleep. If you do, you cut into your health.

Ten hacks for a better night's sleep

As we have seen, improving your sleep can not only improve your diet, but also affect your mood. My sleep problem in my younger days was caused by a variety of factors, including eating (and drinking) late, going to bed at random times, not unwinding before bed (eg, looking at screens) and having bright lights on in my room. Now that I understand its importance, I avoid all these things. Here are my ten top tips for getting more – and better – sleep:

1. Set a regular bedtime

2. Reduce processed foods

3. Eliminate alcohol

4. Eat kiwis

5. Eat high-magnesium foods

6. Don't eat near bedtime

7. Avoid caffeine

8. Limit blue light at night

9. Use candlelight

10. Keep it cool

Set a regular bedtime

Going to bed at a set time both on weekdays and at weekends is important. If your body has just got used to five days of sleeping at a certain time and then at the weekend you throw it a curveball by staying up much later, you aren't going to get quality sleep. And sleep is not like a bank loan that you can 'pay back' by staying in bed the next morning. Sleep is one the most important processes of the body and it needs to be regular. Your body runs like clockwork and will function much better when you have a set bedtime.

Reduce processed foods

Processed foods such as chocolate bars, biscuits, cakes and sweet desserts can all increase your blood sugar levels. This can prevent you falling asleep, especially if you consume them close to your bedtime (see below).

White bread, white pasta, white rice, sauces containing sugars and even some tropical fruit will all give you a spike in your blood sugar compared with their healthier alternatives (containing complex carbs):

brown bread, wholegrain pasta and bulgur wheat or quinoa instead of rice.

Eliminate alcohol

Many of us have a 'nightcap' believing that it will help us sleep. In fact, it has the opposite effect. Alcohol is a drug that interrupts your sleep, causing you to wake during the night and leaving you feeling unrefreshed, no matter how long you spend in bed. You will not remember these small disturbances (waking up in the night) as you are asleep, but alcohol prevents you from getting quality REM sleep – the deepest state of your sleep. Yes, even organic wine, which I'm partial to…

Eat kiwis

These fruits have the ability to get the body to produce melatonin, which aids sleep. Kiwis also contain vitamin C and antioxidants, but also natural sugars – which is why you shouldn't eat them just before going to bed. I also eat them with cinnamon to control my blood sugar levels and prevent a spike, as cinnamon is one of the top five antioxidant spices that reduce stress on the body (see Chapter 8). As a soft fruit, kiwi can be treated with both pesticides and herbicides, so is best eaten organic as excess toxins in the body can prevent you from falling into a deep sleep.

Eat high-magnesium foods

Magnesium is used by the body in numerous different processes. Relaxing the muscles is one of the main ones, which is why foods high in magnesium will help you sleep. Examples of magnesium-rich foods are kale, spinach, broccoli, chard, black and kidney beans, chickpeas and cacao powder. Just 100g of chard or spinach contains nearly 20% of your recommended daily intake of magnesium. Try sprinkling cacao over a yoghurt with two kiwis and cinnamon as a dessert and see how well you sleep!

Don't eat near bedtime

Digesting food is one of the most taxing and stressful jobs for the body, especially if you have a big plate of red meat that the body must break down into its simplest form (amino acids). This will negatively affect your sleep (another reason to add more plant-based protein to your diet) by taking your body's focus away from unwinding, which is not what you want in the evening.

I recommend a minimum of two, if not three, hours between finishing eating and going to bed. If you do need to eat something after that, make sure it's something light like a yoghurt. Instead of going out for late evening meals with friends or partners, go for early-bird menus; they are not just cheaper, they are also better for your sleep.

Avoid caffeine

Some people can't live without it, but it's worth noting that caffeine can stay in your system for more than ten hours. Caffeine is a stimulant, which is why we drink it: to wake us up and make us alert. I use a different stimulus such as maca power as a hot drink in the morning or at lunch. Green tea and mushroom tea are other alternatives that have less caffeine than coffee. If you must have coffee, make sure your last one is at lunchtime so that it doesn't affect your sleep that night.

Limit blue light at night

This is something I was sceptical about until I tried it. Blue light is what comes from computer, tablet and phone screens and prevents the body from producing melatonin.[60] Melatonin helps with sleep, so removing screens or using blue light-blocking glasses (with an orange tinge) limits the effect of the light from digital screens. This is something I do religiously if I must use a screen before bed. This will leave your body to relax naturally and produce melatonin instead of taking expensive supplements, which sometimes don't even work.

Use candlelight

This may seem primitive, but in fact it was quite normal less than a hundred years ago. Since the advent of electric light, we have come so far away from what we were designed to do: go to bed when it's dark and get up when it's light, as nature intended. Using candles in the late evening reduces the amount of artificial light you are exposing your eyes to, to an absolute minimum. It can also create a romantic ambience! Even the light emitted by a standard lightbulb contains blue light, which increases alertness. The red light emitted by a candle or fire (which I light in the winter for both light and heat) doesn't affect your circadian rhythm, ie, your body's twenty-four-hour internal clock. Using candles will also save on electricity bills so that you have more money to buy local, fresh organic food.

A final point on candles is that getting naturally-made candles will reduce your exposure to potentially harmful chemicals. Standard paraffin wax is derived from petroleum and can contain various toxins and carcinogens. Organic waxes such as soy wax or bees-wax are an easy way to avoid risking exposure to such chemicals.

Keep it cool

The temperature of your body is another important factor affecting sleep that is often overlooked. Your core temperature must decrease by 1°C to initiate sleep. This happens naturally when light is reduced and melatonin is increased, but this effect is coun-teracted by the high-tech world we live in, centrally heated homes and even heated car seats.

You will find it easier to fall asleep in a cooler room than a room that is too hot. 18.5°C is the optimal room temperature for the average person. Even if our bedrooms are cool, we often have too many blankets and duvets, pyjamas with fluffy sheep on them, socks, electric blankets… Our bodies then have difficulty dropping their core temperature – particularly if our hands and feet are 'insulated'. When your body is tired, it starts expelling heat, which it radiates from three main areas: your hands, feet and face. These all contain a lot of blood vessels close to the skin, which come into contact with the air. A typical sign that the body is tired is a red face. It is not just a coincidence that many people wash their face before going to bed. Grounding with bare feet on cold tiles can aid sleep too.

Sunlight

There is one thing that we cannot live without and that is the sun. Without it, plants would not grow, bees would not exist and we would die. Lack of sun can lead to diabetes, hormone imbalance, acne and a poorly functioning thyroid, which can prevent weight loss.[61]

Sunlight is energy; it is food. When we think about food, we typically only think of what we eat, but what is the food of our food? Sunlight. What we eat is a secondary source of energy. Why is it that you don't feel as hungry on a hot day as on a cold day? When you get sunlight, especially on your face in the early morning, this reduces your hunger hormone, ghrelin. (This makes early morning sunlight exposure more attractive if you're trying to shed a few pounds.) Another reason that we don't feel as hungry on a warm day is because the body needs less energy to keep itself warm.

All through history, the sun has been used to improve health and even to treat open wounds. Clinics in ancient Greece used it to cure anaemia (due to poor iron in the blood) and bone deformity, later labelled rickets (due to low levels of vitamin D), as well as injuries. While writing this book I nearly lost a finger in a work accident and used the power of the sun to help heal the deep wound.

We are spending increasing amounts of time indoors and filling our homes with 'comforts' that make us want to stay in rather than go out. Natural light is often replaced with some kind of artificial light. We wake up in a closed room; get into a car to drive to work, where we spend all day staring at a laptop under electric lights; go to gym, where we exercise in a climate-controlled room and then go back home, where we spend any remaining daylight hours watching flickering lights from a TV. If we do venture out, we wear so many clothes, creams and make-up that we don't get the full benefit of what the sun has to offer.

And the sun does have a lot to offer. Sunlight is free and one of the few things left 100% uncontaminated. Sunshine is the superfood we don't need to eat.

One of the most important 'supplements' anyone can take is sunlight. In fact, the body cannot function properly without sunlight. Most of us start to feel seasonal affective disorder (SAD) when we don't get enough sun. SAD is caused by a lack of sunlight, so is more common in winter when the days are shorter, as well as in northern countries such as Norway and Finland, where the sun hardly even comes above the horizon in the winter months.

As a society, we are constantly under stress or feeling anxious. Depression is becoming increasingly common and the companies selling anti-depressants are making pots of money, but taking pills to become happy is like putting a sticking plaster over a gaping wound. A far better solution is to switch from an indoor lifestyle to an outdoor one and reap the benefits of natural sunlight:

1. **It detoxifies the body.** Sunlight is a natural anti-bacterial. When you are exposed to sunlight, full-spectrum light (which has all the colours of the rainbow) penetrates your skin, then your veins and, finally, your blood. This removes unwanted toxins from the blood. After as little as ten minutes' exposure to sunlight, most people's

urine turns yellow, which is a sign that toxins are being released from the body.

2. **It improves skin health.**[62] It improves skin health by opening up your pores and making you sweat. Your skin contains thousands of little pores that can become clogged with dirt, causing spots, and in severe cases, acne. Sunlight attracts vitamins and minerals, including vitamins C, D and E and omega-3, to the areas of the skin that it hits. The first sign of good overall health is your skin.

3. **It produces 'happy hormones'.** Sunshine helps to produce serotonin and dopamine to reduce anxiety and depression.[63] One of the reasons sunshine makes us happy (besides the fact that it dries washing on the line) is that it helps the body convert tryptophan (found in eggs, fish and animal livers, pumpkin seeds and oats) into serotonin, the happy hormone. Sunlight also improves blood flow. This leads to a greater amount of that brain-boosting protein, so if you have an exam or presentation coming up, you now have the perfect excuse to lie in the sun!

4. **It reduces pain and speeds up recovery from injuries.**[64] Sunlight reduces pain and speeds up recovery by increasing blood flow.

5. **It improves our ability to learn and retain information.**[65] The rays from the sun penetrate your eyes (the gateway to the brain), improving attention, memory and sight.

6. It increases nutrient absorption and lowers cholesterol.[66]

Vitamin D

Vitamin D is aptly nicknamed the sunshine vitamin. When your bare skin is exposed to sunlight, your cholesterol (found in your skin and blood) produces vitamin D, which is stored in your liver. The more vitamin D that is made, the lower your cholesterol can be. 'Sunshine' and 'cholesterol' are both demonised words (as the saying goes, you *can* have too much of a good thing...), but neither is intrinsically bad for you. It's all a matter of balance and getting the right amount of both, and cholesterol is needed to make vitamin D from sunlight.

There are, of course, foods such as oily fish (mackerel, sardines and salmon), egg yolks, mushrooms and offal (an acquired taste) that contain vitamin D. Your daily vitamin D requirement is 2,000-3,000 IU[67] and these foods would have to be consumed daily to hit that target. There are also vitamin D pills. Cod-liver oil is a supplement that is often recommended for getting vitamin D as well as essential omega-3 fat, but nothing beats what Mother Nature can provide. Depending on the intensity of the sunlight, twenty to thirty minutes' exposure can give you your daily requirement of vitamin D. Why waste money on pills when you can get all the vitamin D you need for free directly from the principal source: the sun?

What exactly does vitamin D do? It can affect mood, immune system, blood flow, brain function and skin condition – which pretty much covers you top-to-toe. If you don't get enough vitamin D, your body will absorb calcium less well. Calcium is, of course, required for strong bones and teeth, but it also helps maintain muscle. Most importantly, perhaps, vitamin D boosts your immune system, helping you to stay healthy, which is key for avoiding flu, viruses or other immune-affecting illnesses.

How much sun do we need?

How much sunlight should we get, when and how? We've been told that the sun is powerful and dangerous. Both are correct, but we focus so much on the negatives that we often overlook the positives. It is the light from the sun, not the heat, that we need, and the idea is to get more of the right type of sunlight. The best times to get it are in the morning or the late evening, when the sun is not too hot.

The required duration of exposure is slightly different for everyone due to their skin pigment and location, but approximately fifteen minutes on your front and fifteen minutes on your back is good for you, particularly if you are trying to reduce back acne or suffer from lower back pain – but anything is better than nothing.

Sunbathing with the sunlight hitting your bare skin has maximum benefits (you don't have to be completely naked, especially if you have nosy neighbours). Anywhere will do (though a beach is nice…): your back garden, a balcony or roof – even indoors. I often sit inside my house with my double doors wide open as I sit on a striped red and white sunchair my mam gave me. Ireland isn't that warm most of the time! 'Sunbathing' through windows is not as effective (as the full spectrum of the sunlight doesn't come through the glass), so open a window to get the full benefits if you have that option in your office or workplace.

Tips for getting more sunlight

1. Let daylight into your house and workplace.

2. Change your exercise to outdoors, if possible. If you must use gym equipment, at least do your cardio outside.

3. Grow your own fruit and veg.

4. Go outside during your work-breaks.

5. Watch the sun rise and/or set.

What about sunscreen?

Sunscreen can, of course, prevent the damaging effects of too much direct sunshine, but it also prevents your body making vitamin D and the chemicals in the product are absorbed into your skin tissues when your pores open up in the sun. This is why I recommend getting your 'doses' of sunlight in the morning and evening, when the sun is at its least powerful. Harsh sun at midday, which can cause burning, is never advised (which is why people in hot countries such as Spain, Italy and Mexico have a siesta during the hottest part of the day; pity the idea hasn't caught on in Ireland...).

Summary

Sleep and sunlight are vitally important for anyone who wants to improve their health. In both cases, it isn't so much a case of quantity as of quality: undisturbed sleep and gentle sunlight are of immeasurable benefit to your body. There are simple ways to get both, and neither will cost you a penny.

12
Personal Development and Happiness

As a small, unsure country boy from the south of Ireland, all I wanted was to be stronger, healthier and happier. It became clear to me that eating quality food and training had big parts to play in achieving this, but I also realised that I needed to mix in my own flavour of positivity to support my journey toward achieving my goals. The final chapter of the book is about adding that 'flavour' to your own life so that you can achieve all that you want to and enjoy the happiness you deserve.

You can't go back in time, but you *can* change the future. Susan Boyle became famous when she sang 'I Dreamed a Dream' from *Les Misérables* at the age of forty-eight. Mary Wesley was seventy-one when she published her first best-selling novel. Never tell yourself that you're too old or that you've missed your chance for success or happiness.

Ten tips for a happier life

Life is a series of small, daily decisions. Right now, wherever you are and whatever you are doing is an accumulated result of those decisions. If you choose better, you will be better, so take time to examine where your values and priorities lie. Here are some tips to assist you on your path to self-development and greater happiness.

Know what you don't want

Some people struggle to define and articulate what they do want, so I try to look at it from a different angle by asking people to write down what it is that they don't want. The need to improve your fitness can be easy to notice from the instant feedback your body usually gives you, but with mental wellbeing it can often be less obvious (for example, a negative relationship or unfulfilling work).

Don't create regrets

If we learn from our mistakes, we won't regret things we've done, but what about things we haven't done?

Twenty years from now, will you look back and be disappointed with your life choices? There are many ways to get to where you want to be. Decide on a path that suits you – one that fits with your goals, your priorities and your lifestyle. The first time I made my own money and had to fend for myself was when I worked in Australia. I wanted to know what to do with the money and my spare time (the norm for my peers was to go out drinking on the weekends). The one person whose opinion really mattered to me was my dad.

I phoned him and asked, 'Dad, what should I do now?' He replied, 'What would you like to do?' His words hit me like a bombshell. What mattered was not what other people wanted me to do, but what I wanted to do. He went on to make this analogy: Doing what others want (or expect) you to is like putting on someone else's clothes. They might more or less fit you, and they might look OK on you, but they've been shaped by another person and will never really be yours. The best thing you can do is pick out new clothes for yourself. I love my dad.

Looking at yourself through the eyes of someone you care about can also help to provide a neutral standpoint and give you more objectivity. What advice would you give yourself to prevent future regrets?

Don't overvalue what you don't have (or undervalue what you do)

It's easy to focus on the things we don't have (a flat stomach, not enough money in the bank, etc), but the more you focus on the perceived negatives, the more they consume you. What others have is nearly always not what it seems. For example, your work colleague has outperformed you and earned a promotion. On the surface, it looks like an enviable situation. Behind the scenes, though, they may have worked fifteen-hour shifts for months on end and only spent two nights a week at home with their family, creating domestic challenges. You didn't get the promotion and accompanying paycheque, but you work a standard forty-hour week and devote more time to the things that you care about. Your colleague has something that you want. You have something your colleague wants. Comparing yourself to others is never a good starting point for any life changes. If you want to be happier, make a conscious choice to be grateful and notice and acknowledge the good things in your life: health, family, friends, job satisfaction – things you wouldn't trade for anything in the world.

Adopt a positive mindset

You are what you eat, but you're also what you think, and you can make yourself happier by adopting a positive mindset. In fact, the sooner you start thinking in a positive manner, the better. Things happen twice in life: first in your mind, and then in reality. Negative thoughts and emotions can skew our perspective and damage our sense of self in the long-term. If you look for something positive each day, whatever it is, your focus on it will expand. The more often you repeat your positive thoughts about what you want in your life, the greater the likelihood of them happening.

One way to get into the habit of thinking positively is to either write down or speak the words of positive quotes or sayings. I use positive affirmations daily, and adopting some of your own will help you on your journey. Expressing what you want out loud can also reinforce your ideas and goals. Think of something that you want in your life and say it out loud to yourself in front of a mirror as if you already have it: 'I'm confident, I'm healthy, I'm happy.' The way you phrase a sentence can have a huge effect on the way your brain processes the information. We can complain that blackberries have thorns, or we can rejoice that they produce berries. Negative thoughts are toxic for the body and the mind.

Face challenges

I was fortunate to spend some time at an Organic Agricultural College in Uganda teaching people the basics of being more self-sufficient, including setting out beds for growing vegetables. I divided one class of thirty into pairs and gave each one an area of land to prepare, but one pair had a problem.

There was a large stone bang in the middle of their bed. They had started to dig it out using their basic tools, but it was the size of a boulder. One of the students, Paul, said, 'Mr Power, my father is a wise man. He told me to always remember that something that cannot speak cannot defeat us.' It was too heavy to lift. In the 40°C (104°F) heat, with sweat rolling down my back, I was stumped. Then Paul suggested that we push the boulder as far as we could in one direction and then place small rocks under it. By repeatedly pushing the boulder onto the smaller rocks, we were eventually able to roll the gigantic obstacle out of the bed. 'Something that cannot speak cannot defeat us.'

Give to others

The first person I trained was a woman whose goal was to lose weight. She texted me to say that not only were her clothes fitting better, but she was confident and proud of the fact that she had reached her fitness goal. It gave me enormous pleasure to be involved in someone else's life-changing journey and the experience inspired me to want to help more people. Everybody can help somebody. Whatever set of skills you have, sharing it with others will bring great satisfaction, so start doing it now. Coach a sport you play in your local club, volunteer to help people learn to read, or buddy up with someone learning a new language. Even doing something as simple as asking someone how they are at a time when they need to talk can be of immeasurable benefit – to you as well as to them. You will always get more from helping others.

Be disciplined

Some days will harder than others and there are certain times of the day when we have more willpower than others, but discipline is an important aspect of self-development. I recommend doing your most important (or least enjoyable) task first thing in the morning. When you get up, you have optimal levels of discipline. This is why some people prefer working out at the beginning of the day: they get their most important tasks done before their workday even starts. When you complete your most difficult task early in the day, you're set up for smoother sailing for the rest of the day. I committed to writing this book first thing every morning. This was challenging, because I had to make the time to write before my workday started. Over time, my morning writing schedule became part of my routine and it was easier to get into the groove. Whatever area you want to improve upon, make it your priority.

An extremely effective approach which helped me to develop discipline is a strategy developed by Darren Hardy in his book, *The Compound Effect: Jumpstart Your Income, Your Life, Your Success*.[68] The 'compound effect' means taking a series of small actions to result in much greater changes and rewards. In fact, this concept helped me write this book. I made myself accountable to write every day by placing €1 in a jar every time I sat down to put pen to paper.

You can do this with your training, too. Using coins is very visual way to track your progress and see that things are adding up. Over time, small incremental improvements will lead to extraordinary results. Self-improvement is a process: day by day, week by week, month by month and year by year.

The compound effect concept has also helped me to slow down. I have a Type A personality and find myself continually wanting to do more and more, but over time I've realised that life is a marathon, not a sprint. Running at top speed all the time leads to burnout further down the line.

The compound effect will help you be more disciplined. People often see the word 'discipline' in a negative light, yet it is actually positive and essential for moving in the right direction toward your goals. When you are self-disciplined (the key word being self), you can become successful in any area of life. Remember that discipline comes from within and is something that you must fine tune over time. You're not born with discipline; you develop it with practice.

Accept support

So much of the knowledge that I now have was passed on to me by coaches and other mentors. With their knowledge and experience, coaches can shorten your own learning curve. Mentors and coaches want the best for you and have the ability to put the information in a way that best serves you. Everyone needs support in different forms and at different times during their lives. Associating with people who are successful (however you define that) in what they do will have a positive effect on how you approach your own work, life and relationships. Spend time with a variety of people who bring out the best in you and try to learn from them.

Practise gratitude

Gratitude is a powerful thing and in practising gratitude, you shift your focus and energy away from negative thoughts. When you are appreciative and grateful, you will undoubtedly feel happier and attract better things into your life. It's also important to appreciate and acknowledge the time and effort anyone has invested in you. (The first people that come to mind is our parents or carers, followed by our immediate family and friends.)

Avoid negative people

When tomato plants are left to grow close together, they develop bad habits. They become lazy and start to lean on each other, so they don't reach their individual potential. When this happens, you need to either separate the plants or pot them in a bigger pot so they can develop and grow properly. The same applies to humans. If we hang around with the same people for too long, we can develop bad habits and become lazy, not thriving as we might have if we had given ourselves space to grow in our own way. If people are being negative towards you and the positive life you are currently living, stand up for yourself or move on to people who support you. You are not a tree; you are not rooted in the position you are currently in.

You can put individuals into two main groups: people who give you energy, and people who take it away. We all know work colleagues, classmates, relatives, friends that give off negative vibes. We also know others who give off positive vibes, are generally upbeat and happy and put you in a good mood. If you limit the amount of time spent with people who bring you down and bring you to their level of unhappiness and increase the amount of time spent with people who bring positive energy, you will become better version of yourself.

There is a false belief that everything needs to be perfect for happiness to be possible. This often happens when you compare yourself with others. Instead, compare yourself with who you were yesterday. If you choose to improve yourself in whatever you have today, aiming to be a little bit better again tomorrow, then you are going in the right direction.

Setting goals

Setting clear, specific goals is a sure-fire way to achieve positive personal development. When you have a goal in mind and consciously choose to write it down, it becomes visible, clear and tangible. It helps you focus on your specific targets and see the steps necessary to achieve them, and you can more readily see your progress, keeping you motivated and focused. People who write things down are nine times more success-ful than those who don't.[69]

Making thoughts real

A dream written down becomes a goal. A goal broken down into steps becomes a plan. A plan backed by action becomes reality. When writing down your goals, be sure to list smaller, interim or short-term goals as well as major, long-term goals. If you want to build a fire, you need big pieces of timber, but you also need kindling. If you start building the fire with the big pieces, it will be difficult to get it going. If you start with the kindling and then add the bigger pieces of timber, the fire will get burning faster and will be hotter and last longer.

Working in a linear way

Following a line is more logical and straightforward than a path full of twists and turns. In horticulture, you can train a fruit tree to follow a wire. It's a slow process. The tree barely moves in twelve months, but apple trees can live anywhere from fifty to eighty years. Each year the branches grow a little bit, and as they do, you train them to follow the wires. You have to drill holes and put up posts, tightening the wires when they get slack due to the weight of apples. After five to six years, maintaining the wire becomes an easy task because you've done all the hard work. The wire is neat and tidy, and the trees are growing well.

We are not unlike fruit trees. If we clearly lay out where we want to go, the way and the endpoint are easier to visualise and achieve. Of course, it's still possible to reach your destination without setting goals – it's just easier to get there if your path is clear and direct.

Creating a goals board

A goals board (or vision board) serves as clear visualisation of your goals and the steps required to get there. You may find it more effective than a written list (I know I do). It can be beneficial to split your goals into areas you want to improve in, for example:

1. Physical and mental health

2. Income/Wealth

3. Relationships

4. Overall personal fulfilment

Under these individual headings, place visual items (pictures, quotes, etc) of exactly what you want from each one. Aim big and don't undersell yourself. Being ambitious is important because goals are meant to be challenging. Shoot for the moon. Even if you miss, you'll end up among the stars, which is still a pretty nice place to be! Visualising your goals and steps and putting them in a place where you can see them every day is essential.

When making your goals board, create separate areas for short- and long-term goals. For example, you can make big fitness strides in a short period of about six to eight weeks, but improvement in overall health requires a lifestyle change, so longer-term goals are important, too. First set your long-term goals (eg, a five-year plan) and then 'reverse-engineer' to set annual, monthly, weekly and daily goals.

Verbalising the items on your goals board while looking in the mirror will reinforce your goals until you begin to believe them. The process of incorporating small changes each day will have a huge effect on where and what you get in the long-term, but believing in yourself is one of the first steps.

Hard work beats talent (when talent doesn't work hard)

When growing up, I was never the most skilled at anything. I was lightweight, a poor student with a learning difficulty and crap with the ladies, so my confidence was low. Sports and exercise did come a bit more easily to me. I wasn't the most talented sportsman, but I could readily see the improvement that came from putting in an effort. I first realised that hard work beats talent when I went to secondary school. I was on every sports team (hurling, soccer, athletics, chess, etc) throughout my six years of schooling for two reasons. First, I loved sports. Second, the more teams I was on, the more likely I was to spend time out of class attending training and matches. I was always there, even if it was lashing rain or the sun was splitting the rocks, but more often than not, I was a sub (and a low-ranked one at that).

I went through the first five years of school without once starting on the hurling team, my favourite sport until one of our players injured his finger and was unable to make the final fifteen for the upcoming match – and it was a final. I got the start – I couldn't believe it! The game was brilliant. In the first five minutes, the ball came in high. The goalkeeper batted it out and I flicked it into the goal. It was an electric feeling. There were probably fewer than fifty people watching, but it felt like a thousand, all celebrating my goal with me. We lost that game, but that didn't matter. I had progressed from being one of the least likely players to be selected for the starting team to scoring in a final due to hard work, perseverance and, of course, a good attitude. These things will serve you well in all aspects of life.

Summary

Life is not all pretty rainbows. In fact, in order for a rainbow to occur, it has to rain somewhere. If you are not happy with where you are (physically, mentally or emotionally), you have the power to change. Little things. Regular things. Things that add up to significant increases in your health, fitness, wellbeing and happiness.

To build a wall, you start by laying a single brick, making sure that it's a colour you like, it's in the right place and it's secure. You continue to do this to the best of your ability until, eventually, you have a wall. When you look back at your wall, you will be satisfied with the way it looks. The same applies to the Wall of Life. (This idea came to me while I was writing this book – I can see a brick wall as I look out of my window. Inspiration is everywhere.)

By applying this approach to fitness, a healthy lifestyle and mindset, you can do anything. You have choices with each meal, each opportunity to exercise and each time you face a challenge. These steps all lead to you getting what you want and deserve. In order to achieve these goals, though, you have to put in the work. One brick does not a wall make!

Conclusion

I certainly wasn't always as healthy as I am now. There was a time when it was a routine of mine to get a weekly take-away, but today I'm far from the boy who lived in the south of Ireland with his parents until he was twenty-four years of age thinking that he was no good. My degrees and personal trainer qualification are important credentials, but more important to me is that I practise what I preach, so I devote my time entirely to fitness and health – mine and other people's.

While I was researching and writing this book, my mind changed in some ways regarding what is required for health, but there is one thing I am still sure about: eating whole foods that have been minimally processed is key to optimum health. When it comes to the best diet, the fewer chemicals the better. And fewer chemicals means organic. It's as simple as that. Having a healthier lifestyle is not a question of eliminating processed food, but of replacing it with natural and home-grown alternatives. Too many people want to lose weight any way they can (and some of the methods out there are pretty extreme), but the important thing is to do it in a healthy way.

There is a lot of information readily available on specific diets, typically endorsing or eliminating specific food groups. My approach is to inform people of the benefits of different foods and lifestyle changes, including exercise and movement that will improve their health in the most natural way possible – organic, you could say.

I'm a firm believer in not just going to the dentist when you have a toothache, or to the doctor only when you're sick, or starting training when you're unfit. If you want to improve your overall health, do so now.

No two people are the same when it comes to choosing a diet. Everyone has different dietary requirements, different food preferences and different moral perspectives. The important thing is to pick the foods that best suit you and your lifestyle. Remember that everything you consume affects the person you become. That goes for both foods and information from your environment, so make sure you surround yourself with food and people who will help you progress towards a better version of yourself.

Whatever stage you are in your fitness and health journey, all you are looking for is an improvement. With each task you set out to do, you improve as a person and build in confidence. I hope this book has encouraged you to make lifestyle changes with the goal of living your best life. If, after reading this book, you want to learn more and live a healthier lifestyle then The Colman Power Organic Fitness website is the best place to start.

My Organic Fitness Training Program is a six- to eight-week course that covers all the information covered in this book: foods, exercise routines and advice on reducing inflammation and improving your sleep, leading to an improvement in your overall health. The programme introduces you to chemical-free organic produce, which I recommend including in your diet; just follow the link below.

For more general information on organic fitness or if you are interested in joining the Colman Power Organic Fitness Program, go to: www.colmanpower-organicfitness.com

Notes

1   Seesen, M, et al, 2020. Association between
    organophosphate pesticide exposure and
    insulin resistance in pesticide sprayers and
    non-farmworkers. *International Journal of
    Environmental Research and Public Health*, 17(21),
    p8140.
2   Astrup, A, et al, 2020. Saturated fats and health:
    a reassessment and proposal for food-based
    recommendations: JACC state-of-the-art review.
    Journal of the American College of Cardiology, 76(7),
    pp844–857.
3   Miranda, JM, et al, 2015. Egg and egg-derived
    foods: effects on human health and use as
    functional foods. *Nutrients*, 7(1), pp706–729.
4   Miyazaki, K, et al, 2014. Bifidobacterium
    fermented milk and galacto-oligosaccharides

lead to improved skin health by decreasing phenols production by gut microbiota. *Beneficial Microbes, 5*(2), pp121–128.

5 Bruce-Keller, AJ, et al, 2018. Harnessing gut microbes for mental health: getting from here to there. *Biological Psychiatry, 83*(3), pp214–223.

6 Bulsiewicz, W, *Fiber Fueled: The Plant-Based Gut Health Program for Losing Weight, Restoring Your Health, and Optimizing Your Microbiome* (Penguin, 2022).

7 Lin, WT, et al, 2020. The association between sugar-sweetened beverages intake, body mass index, and inflammation in US adults. *International Journal of Public Health, 65*(1), pp45–53.

8 Ursin, R, 2002. Serotonin and sleep. *Sleep Medicine Reviews, 6*(1), pp55–67.

9 Nettleton, JE, et al, 2016. Reshaping the gut microbiota: Impact of low calorie sweeteners and the link to insulin resistance. *Physiology & Behavior, 164*, pp488–493.

10 Zhu, C, et al, 2018. Carbon dioxide (CO2) levels this century will alter the protein, micronutrients, and vitamin content of rice grains with potential health consequences for the poorest rice-dependent countries. *Science Advances, 4*(5), eaaq1012.

11 European Commission, 2019. The Organic Logo. https://ec.europa.eu/info/food-farming-fisheries/farming/organic-farming/organic-logo_en [accessed 6 April 2022]

12 Seneff, S, *Toxic Legacy: How the Weedkiller Glyphosate Is Destroying Our Health and the Environment* (Chelsea Green Publishing, 2021).

13 Yadav, IC. and Devi, NL, 2017. Pesticides classification and its impact on human and environment. *Environmental Science and Engineering, 6*, pp140–158.

14 Hurtado-Barroso, S, et al, 2019. Organic food and the impact on human health. *Critical Reviews in Food Science and Nutrition, 59*(4), pp704–714.

15 Caldeira, C, et al, 2019. Quantification of food waste per product group along the food supply chain in the European Union: A mass flow analysis. *Resources, Conservation and Recycling, 149*, pp479–488.

16 Popa, ME, et al, 2019. Organic foods contribution to nutritional quality and value. *Trends in Food Science & Technology, 84*, pp15–18.

17 Seneff, S, *Toxic Legacy: How the Weedkiller Glyphosate Is Destroying Our Health and the Environment* (Chelsea Green Publishing, 2021).

18 Huber, M, et al, 2011. Organic food and impact on human health: Assessing the status quo and prospects of research. *NJAS: Wageningen Journal of Life Sciences, 58*(3-4), pp103–109.

19 Barański, M, et al, 2014. Higher antioxidant and lower cadmium concentrations and lower incidence of pesticide residues in organically grown crops: a systematic literature review and meta-analyses. *British Journal of Nutrition, 112*(5), pp794–811.

20 Charron, CS, et al, 2015. A single meal containing raw, crushed garlic influences expression of immunity- and cancer-related genes in whole blood of humans. *The Journal of Nutrition, 145*(11), pp2448–2455.

21 Crinnion, WJ, 2010. Organic foods contain higher levels of certain nutrients, lower levels of pesticides, and may provide health benefits for the consumer. *Alternative Medicine Review, 15*(1).

22 Available on my website: www. colmanpowerorganicfitness.com

23 Bruno, E, et al, 2016. Adherence to WCRF/ AICR cancer prevention recommendations and metabolic syndrome in breast cancer patients. *International Journal of Cancer, 138*(1), pp237–244.

24 Palozza, Paola, et al, 2012. Effect of lycopene and tomato products on cholesterol metabolism. *Annals of Nutrition and Metabolism, 61*(2), pp126–134.

25 Kang, JH, et al, 2009. Vitamin E, vitamin C, beta carotene, and cognitive function among women with or at risk of cardiovascular disease: The Women's Antioxidant and Cardiovascular Study. *Circulation, 119*(21), pp2772–2780.

26 Kalt, W, et al, 2020. Recent research on the health benefits of blueberries and their anthocyanins. *Advances in Nutrition, 11*(2), pp224–236.

27 Mayoclinic.org, 2022. *Cold sore - Diagnosis and treatment - Mayo Clinic.* www.mayoclinic.org/ diseases-conditions/cold-sore/diagnosis-treatment/drc-20371023 [accessed 27 January 2022]

28 Carvalho, AM, et al, 2020. Phytol, a Chlorophyll component, produces anti-hyperalgesic, anti-inflammatory, and antiarthritic effects: possible NFκB pathway involvement and reduced levels of the proinflammatory cytokines TNF-α and IL-6. *Journal of Natural Products*, *83*(4), pp1107–1117.

29 The EWG is American activist group that specialises in research and advocacy in the areas of agricultural subsidies, toxic chemicals, drinking water pollutants and corporate accountability. EWG is a non-profit organization (www.ewg.org).

30 Lotti, F, and Maggi, M, Sexual dysfunction and male infertility. *Nature Reviews Urology*, *15*(5), pp287–307.

31 Roncero-Ramos, I, and Delgado-Andrade, C, 2017. The beneficial role of edible mushrooms in human health. *Current Opinion in Food Science*, *14*, pp122–128.

32 *Science Daily*, May 2017. Nutritional properties of mushrooms are better preserved when they are grilled or microwaved. www.sciencedaily.com/releases/2017/05/170519083817.htm [accessed 15 March 2022]

33 Systematic Review of Phenolic Compounds in Apple Fruits: Compositions, Distribution, Absorption, Metabolism, and Processing Stability. *Journal of Agricultural and Food Chemistry*, *69*(1), pp7–27 doi: 10.1021/acs.jafc.0c05481.

34 Kent, K, et al, 2017. Consumption of anthocyanin-rich cherry juice for 12 weeks improves memory and cognition in older adults with mild-to-moderate dementia. *European Journal of Nutrition, 56*, pp333–341.

35 Cockayne, S, et al, 2006. Vitamin K and the prevention of fractures: systematic review and meta-analysis of randomized controlled trials. *Archives of Internal Medicine, 166*(12), pp1256–1261.

36 Holford, P, *Optimum Nutrition For The Mind* (Piatkus, 2010).

37 Greger, M and Stone, G, *How Not To Die: Discover the Foods Scientifically Proven To Prevent and Reverse Disease* (Pan Macmillan, 2016).

38 Benzie, IF and Wachtel-Galor, *Herbal Medicine: Biomolecular and Clinical Aspects* (CRC Press, 2011).

39 Karakol, P, and Kapi, E, 'Use of Selected Antioxidant-Rich Spices and Herbs in Foods'. In *Antioxidants* by Waisundara, V, (IntechOpen, 2021), pp383–406.

40 Maghbooli, M, et al, 2014. Comparison between the efficacy of ginger and sumatriptan in the ablative treatment of the common migraine. *Phytotherapy Research, 28*(3), pp412–415.

41 Jenabi, E, 2013. The effect of ginger for relieving of primary dysmenorrhoea. *Journal of Pakistan Medical Association, 63*(1), pp8–10.

42 Akazawa, N, et al, 2012. Curcumin ingestion and exercise training improve vascular endothelial

function in postmenopausal women. *Nutrition Research*, 32(10), pp795–799.

43 Shajib, MS, et al, 2017. Diverse effects of gut-derived serotonin in intestinal inflammation. *ACS Chemical Neuroscience*, 8(5), pp920–931.

44 Mekonnen, MM and Hoekstra, AY, 2010. Water footprint of crop and animal products: a comparison. http://waterfootprint.org/en/water-footprint/product-water-footprint/water-footprint-crop-and-animal-products [accessed 27 January 2022].

45 Soliman, GA, 2018. Dietary cholesterol and the lack of evidence in cardiovascular disease. *Nutrients*, 10(6), p780.

46 Temple, NJ, Supplements to Our Diets: Navigating a Minefield, pp435–445. In *Nutrition Guide for Physicians and Related Healthcare Professions* (Humana Press, 2022).

47 Meissner, HO, et al, 2006. Hormone-balancing effect of pre-gelatinized organic Maca (Lepidium peruvianum Chacon): (III) clinical responses of early-postmenopausal women to Maca in double blind, randomized, placebo-controlled, crossover configuration, outpatient study. *International Journal of Biomedical Science: IJBS*, 2(4), p375.

48 Yeung, KS, et al, 2018. Herbal medicine for depression and anxiety: A systematic review with assessment of potential psycho-oncologic relevance. *Phytotherapy Research*, 32(5), pp865–891.

49 Wang, Y, et al, 2007. Maca: An Andean crop with multi-pharmacological functions. *Food Research International*, 40(7), pp783–792.

50 Večeřa, R, et al, 2007. The influence of maca (Lepidium meyenii) on antioxidant status, lipid and glucose metabolism in rat. *Plant Foods for Human Nutrition*, 62(2), pp59–63.

51 Duhigg, C, *The Power of Habit: Why We Do What We Do in Life and Business* (Random House, 2012).

52 Mikkelsen, K, and Apostolopoulos, V, 2019. Vitamin B1, B2, B3, B5, and B6 and the immune system, pp115–125. In *Nutrition and Immunity* (Springer, 2019).

53 Monteiro, BC, et al, 2017. Relationship between brain-derived neurotrofic factor (Bdnf) and sleep on depression: a critical review. *Clinical Practice and Epidemiology in Mental Health: CP & EMH*, 13, p213.

54 National Institutes of Health, 2016. Magnesium fact sheet for health professionals. https://ods.od.nih.gov/factsheets/Magnesium-HealthProfessional [accessed 26 April 2022].

55 Engin, A, and Engin, A, 2021. Risk of Alzheimer's Disease and Environmental Bisphenol A exposure. *Current Opinion in Toxicology*, 25, pp36–41.

56 Scoon, GS, et al, 2007. Effect of post-exercise sauna bathing on the endurance performance of competitive male runners. *Journal of Science and Medicine in Sport*, 10(4), pp259–262.

57 Brueck, H, 2019, A fitness guru who goes by
    'Iceman' says exposure to extreme temperatures
    is a lifesaving third pillar of physical health,
    (Insider, 2019), www.businessinsider.com/
    iceman-wim-hof-dutch-technique-science-2019-
    1?r=US&IR=T [accessed 15 March 2022].

58 Oschman, JL, et al, 2015. The effects of
    grounding (earthing) on inflammation,
    the immune response, wound healing,
    and prevention and treatment of chronic
    inflammatory and autoimmune diseases. *Journal
    of Inflammation Research, 8,* p83.

59 Henst, RH, et al, 2019. The effects of sleep
    extension on cardiometabolic risk factors: A
    systematic review. *Journal of Sleep Research, 28*(6),
    e12865.

60 Shechter, A, et al, 2018. Blocking nocturnal blue
    light for insomnia: A randomized controlled
    trial. *Journal of Psychiatric Research, 96,* pp196–
    202.

61 Pittas, AG, et al, 2006. Vitamin D and calcium
    intake in relation to type 2 diabetes in women.
    Diabetes Care, 29(3), pp650–656.

62 Dakhole, P, and Dakhole, P, 2019. Role of Chitrak
    in the Management of Skin Problem WSR to
    Shwitra. *Journal of Drug Delivery and Therapeutics,
    9*(5), pp213–215.

63 Wang, R, et al, 2019. Cross-sectional associations
    between long-term exposure to particulate
    matter and depression in China: the mediating
    effects of sunlight, physical activity, and

neighborly reciprocity. *Journal of Affective Disorders*, 249, pp8–14.

64 Ubbink, DT, et al, 2015. Evidence-based care of acute wounds: a perspective. *Advances in Wound Care*, 4(5), pp286–294.

65 Zhu, H, et al, 2018. Moderate UV exposure enhances learning and memory by promoting a novel glutamate biosynthetic pathway in the brain. *Cell*, 173(7), pp1716–1727.

66 Grimes, DS, et al, 1996. Sunlight, cholesterol and coronary heart disease. *QJM: An International Journal of Medicine*, 89(8), pp579–590.

67 The amount of vitamin D is given in International Units (IU). 2,000 IU is equivalent to 50 micrograms.

68 Hardy, D, *The Compound Effect: Jumpstart Your Income, Your Life, Your Success* (Perseus, 2012).

69 Canfield, J, *The Success Principles: How To Get From Where You Are To Where You Want To Be* (Harper, 2005).

Acknowledgements

There are two very special people I'd like to mention: Brian Kean and Klause Laitenberger – both mentors of mine. Brian has helped me both mentally with a stronger mindset, and in my business. Klause was my growing mentor and taught me pretty much everything I know in terms of sowing seeds to organic methods. Mentors or coaches help people shorten their learning curve; it's not to say I would not have got to where I am now without guidance, but it would have taken considerably longer.

I'd also like to acknowledge all the people that I have met along the way, from clients to studies and even people on social media that I chat to all around the world. Life is about experiences and when you meet likeminded people, you will see the difference in yourself. I don't have a TV (partly down to Brian who once asked, 'What's not on it that you couldn't watch on Netflix on your laptop?') and partly from Klause mentioning that 'time is something you cannot get back'; even though he may have meant in sowing seeds terms, I took it as a life metaphor.

Everything you consume reflects the person you become, and that goes for both food and information from people you read or listen to. Make sure you find people who will help create the best version of you.

I have to also thank both my uncle, William Power, who took photos for the cover and Cormac Duffy, my second photographer (yes, I needed two for my big head) who also provided me with a studio to take the high-quality images. But for them, the front cover may have been a set of dumbbells and a bowl of fruit and veg!

My final thanks is for a family member currently based in Melbourne, Australia, who willingly took on the task of proofreading chapter by chapter, right from the start when no one else knew about the book. Thanks, Mary Ann Tobin.

The Author

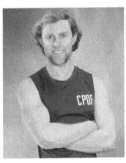

Coming from a country background, I was friends with everyone, but struggled to fit in with any specific group. Not knowing exactly what to do coming out of school, I was lucky enough to be told to do something I thought I would enjoy. For me, that meant growing – in every sense of the word.

Because I'm dyslexic and not particularly academic, it took a lot of grit and determination for me to study. After obtaining a degree in Horticulture and Land Management, I was delighted to achieve a Master's degree in Organic Horticulture (with massive help along the way). The confidence I gained from reaching this goal gave me further fuel in the fire to complete a degree in Education and a qualification in Personal Training.

Setting up my own business to share the knowledge of how to eat healthier and the benefits of exercise was my next goal. Coaching and mentoring people and encouraging them to eat local, fresh organic produce while training is my dream job.

⊕ www.colmanpowerorganicfitness.com

◉ https://open.spotify.com/
show/4xdAsDMSEDnfffSsqN7RRM

▥ Stitcher: www.stitcher.com/show/colman-power

◎ www.instagram.com/
colman_power_organic_fitness/?hl=en

♪ Tik Tok: www.tiktok.com/@
colmanpower?lang=en

🅵 www.facebook.com/colman.power

Lightning Source UK Ltd.
Milton Keynes UK
UKHW021532040722
405349UK00010B/2216